1

THE PATHOLOGY OF SHOCK

JUDITH K. BOBB, RN, BSN

SHOCK

A Nursing Guide

Jacqueline M. Carolan, RN, BSN, CCRN
Head Nurse, Critical Surgical Care/Shock and Trauma Unit
Hahnemann University Hospital, Philadelphia

WRIGHT
Bristol 1986

British Library Cataloguing in Publication Data

Carolan, Jacqueline M.
Shock: a nursing guide.
1. Shock
I. Title
617'.21 RB150.S5
ISBN 0-7236-0879-2

Cover design by Tom Darnsteadt
Cover photograph by Stephen Munz
Interior design by Rachel Geswaldo

ISBN 0-7236-0879-2

John Wright & Sons Ltd, Techno House,
Redcliffe Way, Bristol BS1 6NX, England

Printed in the United States of America

CONTENTS

CONTRIBUTORS

Judith K. Bobb, RN, BSN

Nurse coordinator, Maryland Institute for Emergency Medical Services Systems, Baltimore

Jacqueline M. Carolan, RN, BSN, CCRN

Head nurse, critical surgical care/shock and trauma unit, Hahnemann University Hospital, Philadelphia, Pennsylvania

Gloria Oblouk Darovic, RN, CCRN

Nurse instructor/clinician in critical care, Medical Center Hospital, and lecturer/consultant for American Medical Education, Largo, Florida

LuAnne M. Franco, RN, MSN, CCRN

Clinical nurse specialist, Allen Neurosurgical Associates, Allentown, Pennsylvania

Billie C. Meador, RN, MS, CCRN

Lecturer, baccalaureate nursing program, San Diego State University, San Diego, California

Patricia A. Meehan, RN, MS, CCRN

Clinical nurse specialist in critical care, Westchester County Medical Center, Valhalla, New York

Ann M. Petlin, RN, BSN, CCRN

Staff nurse, medical intensive care unit, Hospital of the University of Pennsylvania, Philadelphia

Georgina Randolph, RN, MBA, MSN

Clinical administrator, Brandywine Dialysis Center, Wilmington, Delaware

Kathleen Scanlon, RN, BSN

Nurse educator, Hahnemann University Hospital, Philadelphia, Pennsylvania

Gloria Sonnesso, RN, MSN, CCRN

Pulmonary clinical specialist, Albert Einstein Medical Center, Northern Division, Philadelphia, Pennsylvania

Rhonda M. Weller, RN, MSN

Nursing instructor, Community Medical Center, Scranton, Pennsylvania

Clareen A. Wiencek, RN, MSN, CCRN

Unit director, medical intensive care, Indiana University Medical Center, Indianapolis

FOREWORD

Increasing numbers of acutely ill and injured patients are surviving because shock has been reversed or prevented. Sophisticated technology and the routine use of invasive as well as noninvasive monitoring devices have made these gains possible. But it's we as nurses, who perform the monitoring and interpret the results, who are truly responsible for successful outcomes.

Bringing patients through shock calls upon all our clinical skills. Preventing shock, however, is even more desirable. "Prevention is the best therapy" is nowhere more true than in shock—and it demands the utmost of our scientific knowledge and bedside vigilance.

When monitoring critically ill patients, we must be able to anticipate problems that might develop but are not yet clinically evident. We must also be able to assess the likelihood of such problems developing, based on our ongoing observations and measurements of vital signs, respiratory sufficiency, fluid status, cardiovascular function, and blood gases, among other clinical parameters. In addition, we must be constantly aware of the short-term and far-reaching effects of our own nursing interventions.

SHOCK: A NURSING GUIDE brings together all these clinical skills with a solid basis of scientific knowledge—the "why" as well as the "how." The first two chapters summarize the basic pathology of shock and the principles of assessment that logically follow. Chapter 3 presents the direct and derived parameters used in monitoring and explains the operation of invasive devices such as the flow-directed balloon catheter. The next several chapters are devoted to the mechanisms, treatment, and nursing implications of the various types of shock—hypovolemic, septic, cardiogenic, neurogenic, and anaphylactic—as well as disseminated intravascular coagulation and renal failure. Temperature and adrenal responses and nutritional needs are the subjects of the final chapters. And don't overlook the appendix, a table of drugs used in critical care.

Jackie Carolan and her contributors are to be commended for putting together this small but useful volume. It should serve the professional needs of all nurses, not just those specializing in critical care. The ultimate beneficiaries will be our patients.

Margaret Van Meter, RN
Clinical Editor, *RN* Magazine

PUBLISHER'S NOTES

Jacqueline M. Carolan, RN, BSN, CCRN, is head nurse on the critical surgical care/shock and trauma unit at Hahnemann University Hospital in Philadelphia, with responsibility for management, budget, and education. She was previously a staff nurse on the same unit—a position that has enabled her to add a practical, "hands-on" perspective to the task of editing SHOCK: A NURSING GUIDE.

Ms. Carolan participates in teaching the intensive care course at Hahnemann University Hospital and has guest-lectured at other institutions on subjects ranging from clinical concepts to ethics.

With Ann M. Petlin, RN, Ms. Carolan is the coauthor of two articles published in *RN* Magazine. She also contributed two chapters to MANAGING THE CRITICALLY ILL EFFECTIVELY, edited by Margaret Van Meter, RN (Medical Economics Books, 1982).

Shock has been defined as "A state in which blood flow to peripheral tissues is inadequate to sustain life."[1] It is a derangement of homeostasis that deprives these tissues of the oxygen and nutrients required to maintain normal metabolism, and it may be due to various causes. In fact, until recently, it was usual to classify this clinical syndrome according to cause. Advances in medical practice and technology have, however, led to a more accurate understanding of shock on the basis of cellular function.

Etiology

The causes of shock include the following traumatic or pathophysiologic insults:

1. *Hemorrhage,* which curtails the blood supply by reducing the blood volume. First in rank among the causes of shock, it is most often due to trauma (Table 1-1).
2. *Burns or dehydration,* which lead to a reduction of the blood's plasma fraction and a decline in total blood volume.
3. *Impaired heart function,* producing a fall in cardiac output.
4. *Overwhelming sepsis,* whose mechanism is less well understood. Septic or toxic shock is believed to include activation of the complement and coagulation systems, mainly by the endotoxins of gram-negative bacteria. (*Escherichia coli* and *Klebsiella* organisms are the most commonly reported causative agents.[2]) The microthrombi thus formed occlude the vessels and, it is believed, lead to maldistribution of the blood volume within the circulatory system. Hypovolemia complicates septic shock by increasing capillary permeability and causing extravasation of fluid out of the vascular compartment.

5. *Diminished sympathetic stimulation,* which may lead to a loss of peripheral vascular resistance, causing dilation of the vascular bed and a decline or fluctuation in blood pressure. This condition is most often seen following spinal cord transection or in association with spinal anesthesia.

Table 1-1. Common Causes of Hemorrhage/Hypovolemia

Trauma
Burns
Anaphylaxis
Gastrointestinal disorders
Anticoagulant therapy
Diuretics
Clotting or bleeding disorders

The microcirculation

Structure and function. The small vessels that supply blood to the tissue cells are the arterioles, capillaries, and venules. Water, nutrients, and respiratory gases are exchanged across the capillaries. These small vessels, made up of a single layer of endothelial cells, have a diameter approximately equal to that of an erythrocyte.

Normal capillary blood flow is regulated by the precapillary arterioles. Unlike capillaries, they constrict or dilate in response to changes in neural regulation, pressure, oxygen demand, or vasoactive substances. In some cases, groups of smooth muscle cells surround the capillaries. These are known as precapillary sphincters and seem to play a major role in the pathophysiology of shock.

Response during shock. The body usually responds to illness or injury by activating the neurohumoral systems. As a result, vascular tone—dominated by the sympathetic division of the autonomic nervous system—is directly increased, as is release of norepinephrine and epinephrine from the adrenal medulla. At first, blood flow remains unchanged; however, when the effective circulating intravascular volume declines, additional vasoconstriction ensues. Precapillary sphincters in skeletal and cardiac muscle, the mesentery, and kidneys constrict, reducing flow to these organs. Still, flow to the heart is maintained, since this organ and the brain are autoregulated (that is, flow is governed by local rather than systemic factors.)

With progressive loss of effective volume, microcirculatory perfusion is reduced. The resulting ischemia and anoxia cause the release of several vasoactive and vasotoxic substances, including bradykinin, prostaglandins, and myocardial depressant factor. In addition, serotonin and histamine may be released from platelets. A common effect of these agents is an increase in capillary permeability, causing fluid to move into the interstitial space and further reducing intravascular volume. Anoxia also stimulates the synthesis and release of prostaglandins and thromboxanes, which exhibit vasoconstrictive effects and can induce platelet aggregation. (Both red cells and platelets can adhere to the walls of the vessels and to each other.) These cell aggregates contribute further to tissue ischemia. Myocardial depressant factor, a polypeptide, appears to be released by the ischemic pancreas. Its actions include negative inotropism, splanchnic vasoconstriction, and depressed phagocytosis.

Cellular changes in shock

The ischemia and hypoxia of shock lead to gradual changes in the function of the intracellular organelles,

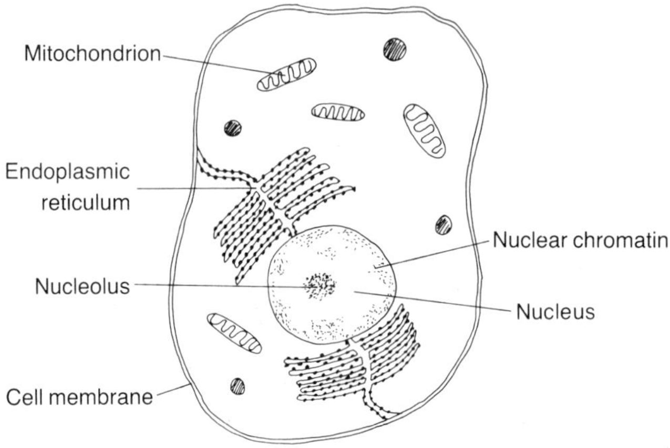

Figure 1-1. Drawing of normal cell.

most notably the plasma membrane, mitochondria, and endoplasmic reticulum (Figure 1-1). These stages have been described in detail.[3] Beginning with the normal cell (stage I), great metabolic defects of water balance, energy production, and ion transport develop over stages II to IV. Irreversible changes characterize stages V through VII (Table 1-2).

The plasma membrane

Structure and function. The cell is separated from its environment by a limiting plasma membrane consisting of a central phospholipid bilayer bound on each side by structural protein, the outer surface of which is coated by polysaccharides. This membrane is believed to be perforated by small pores through which water and some molecules can pass (Figure 1-2).

Water moves freely across the plasma membrane according to its osmotic gradient in the normal cell. Some small molecules and ions diffuse passively or with a carrier. Other ions, though able to penetrate the membrane, are in the main transported actively *against* their respective concentration gradients. In particular, this is true of sodium (Na^+) and potassium (K^+). The separation of ions across the cell membrane serves many essential functions: It helps determine cell shape and movement and is necessary for impulse transmission across the membrane as well as for energy production and protein synthesis. A membrane pump is believed to

Table 1-2. Stages of Cell Injury*

I	Normal cell
II	Hypoxia, loss of ATP Failure of membrane pumps Membrane blebs
III	Mitochondrial condensation Dilation of ER Ion movement
IV	Cellular swelling
V	Cellular swelling Mitochondrial swelling Dense flocculent particles
VI	Intracellular disruption Breaks in plasma membrane
VII	Degradation of cell

*Adapted, with permission, from Trump BF, Berezesky IK, Cowley RA: The cellular and subcellular characteristics of acute and chronic injury with emphasis on the role of calcium. In *Pathophysiology of Shock, Anoxia, and Ischemia* (Trump BF, Cowley RA, eds). Baltimore: Williams & Wilkins, 1982

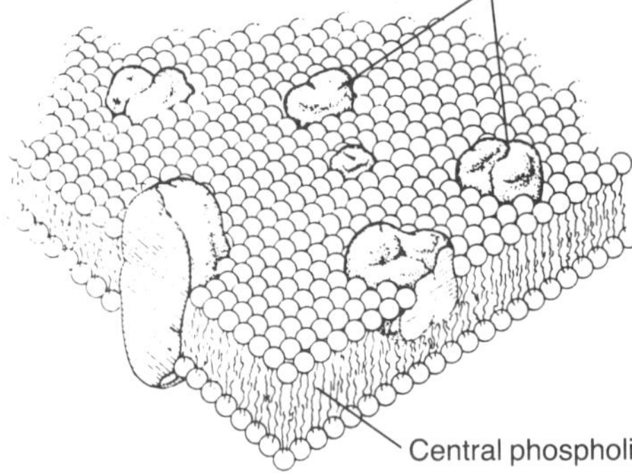

Figure 1-2. Drawing of cell membrane. Reproduced, with permission, from Singer SJ, Nicolson GL: The fluid mosaic model for membrane structure. Science 175:720, 1972.

account for this process. Adenosine triphosphate (ATP), a high-energy compound derived from the metabolism of foodstuffs, is the fuel that drives this pump.

Response during shock. Early morphologic changes in the cell membrane during shock are visible under the electron microscope. Extrusions or blebs of the membrane are formed, and these may break off entirely. A current hypothesis is that this is in some way related to changes in the calcium ion concentration [Ca^{++}].[4] Functional changes in the membrane decrease the activity of the Na^+-K^+ pump. This causes increased permeability to these ions, which now move *along* their concentration gradients. K^+ leaves the cell, and the influx of sodium inside is paralleled by the movement of water. The cell begins to swell.

The mitochondria

Structure and function. Within the cytoplasm, the synthesis of energy in the form of ATP takes place in the

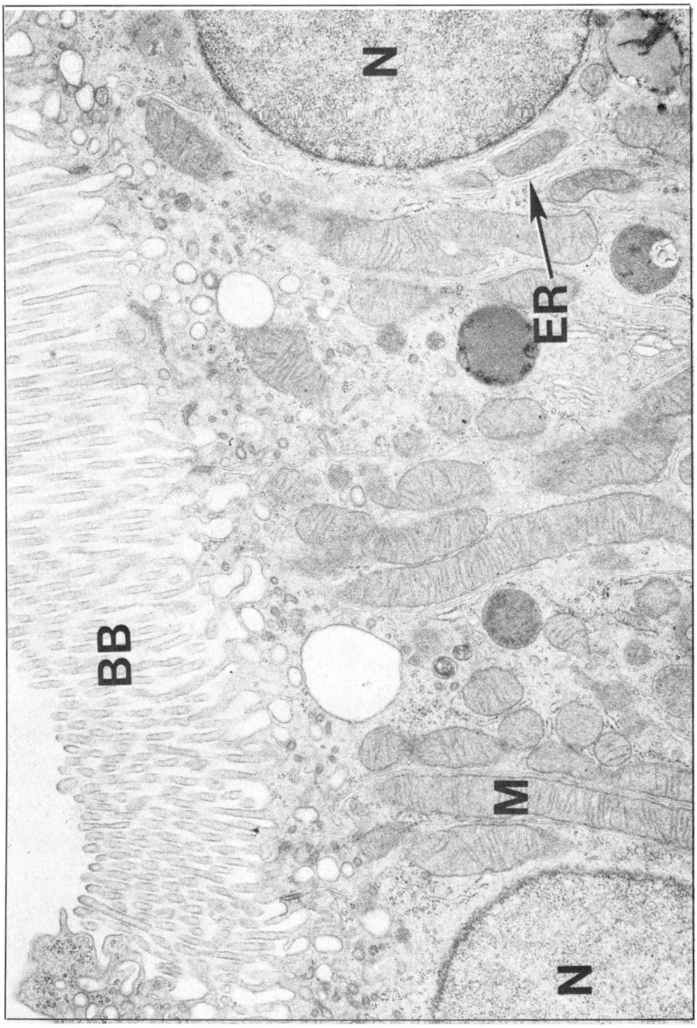

Figure 1-3. Electron micrograph (×8,000) depicting normal cell structure. This cell from a rat kidney shows portions of a normal proximal convoluted tubule. Note elongated mitochondria (M) in orthodox conformation, endoplasmic reticulum (ER), brush border (BB), and nuclei (N). (Electron micrograph courtesy of B. F. Trump, M.D., Department of Pathology, University of Maryland School of Medicine.)

mitochondrion. This organelle consists of an outer, limiting membrane and an inner, invaginated membrane known as the crista (Figure 1-3). The respiratory enzymes are membrane-bound and the enzymes of the citric acid cycle are in the matrix. These enzymes break carbon-chain foods down into carbon dioxide (CO_2) and water, releasing ATP in the process. The number of mitochondria is related to the cell's energy expenditure. There may be as many as 4,000 in a single liver cell.

Response during shock. With ischemia or anoxia, the cell's production of ATP is severely curtailed and its intracellular levels fall. This not only affects the plasma membrane pumps but also alters the sequestration of various ions within the mitochondria themselves.

During shock, the inner membranes of the mitochondria shrink—a process associated with increased sodium and water content. This condensation of the inner membrane also correlates with decreases in K^+ and magnesium and possibly with loss of Ca^{++}.[4] Under the electron microscope, such mitochondria appear dense, and the inner and outer membranes may be seen to have separated. Eventually, the evidence of irreversibility will appear in this organelle.

The mitochondrion also loses the ability to metabolize its nutrients completely. The digestive process is interrupted after glycolysis, the stage at which pyruvate is converted to lactate, giving rise to intracellular as well as extracellular acidosis. Although acidemia is generally considered to be detrimental, it has been suggested that it may prolong the survival of the anoxic cell.[4]

The endoplasmic reticulum

Structure and function. The endoplasmic reticulum (ER) is a tubular or canal-like structure filled with fluid and enclosed by a limiting membrane (Figure 1-3). It has many anastomoses as well as cavities called cisternae. The ER may look granulated when membrane-

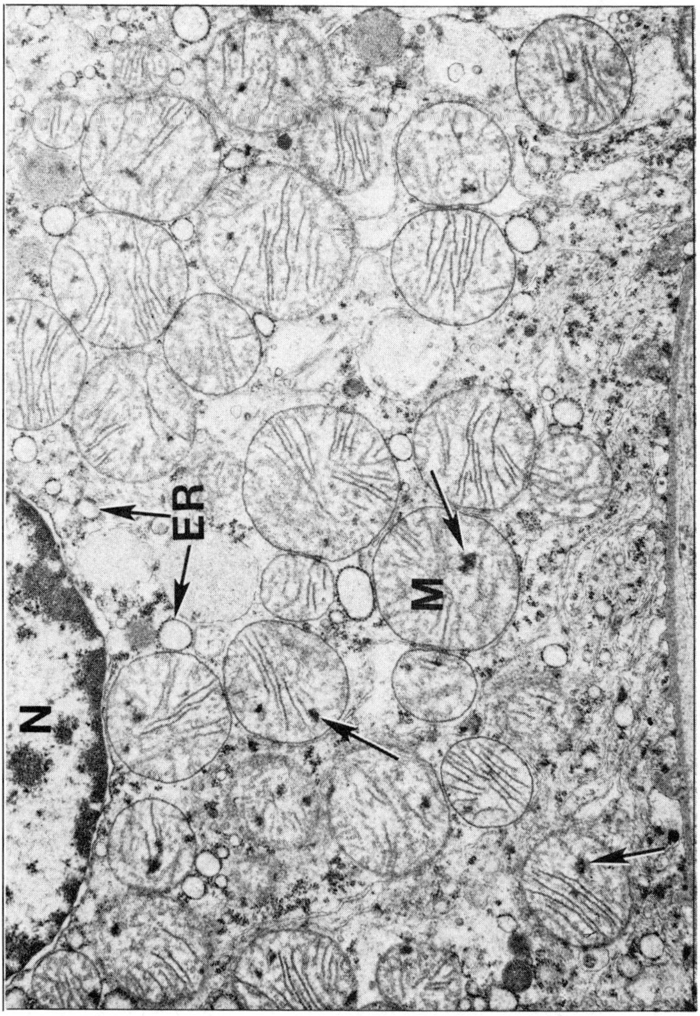

Figure 1-4. Electron micrograph (× 18,000) of cell during shock. This portion of proximal convoluted tubule cell from rat kidney has been subjected to 120 minutes of ischemia in vivo. All mitochondria (M) exhibit marked swelling, and most contain flocculent densities (arrows), the hallmark of irreversibility. Note the nucleus (N) with marginated chromatin and the dilated ER (arrows). (Electron micrograph courtesy of B. F. Trump, M.D., Department of Pathology, University of Maryland School of Medicine.)

bound ribosomes are present. Ribosomes are particles of ribonucleoprotein and are the site of protein synthesis. Synthesized protein, in turn, is secreted into the lumen of the ER for transport.

Smooth ER lacks ribosomes. In skeletal muscle, smooth ER sequesters calcium. In some endocrine glands, it is the site of steroid formation. It may also play a role in the formation of lipids in the liver.

Response during shock. The chief alteration in the ER during shock is dilation. Again, this correlates with influx of sodium, movement of water, and efflux of potassium. Cell water may not always increase, but it is postulated that it is redistributed into the ER.

Point of no return

The point of no return, according to Trump,[3,4] occurs at stage V, when dense, flocculent particles appear in the swollen mitochondria (Figure 1-4). Although the exact nature of these particles is still uncertain, they are believed to be denatured matrix proteins. No therapy, at this point, can keep the cells alive. They undergo disruption and digestion (stage VI) and final degradation (stage VII; see Table 1-2).

Clearly, these changes do not affect every cell with equal speed. Some cells require less oxygen than others and therefore survive longer; others succumb rapidly. In the human, the point of no return is reached in about an hour. After that, attempts to resuscitate the patient are bound to fail.

REFERENCES

1. Berkow R (Ed): *The Merck Manual of Diagnosis and Therapy*, 13th ed. Rahway, NJ: Merck & Co, 1977, p 395

2. Landesman SH, Gorbach SL: Gram negative sepsis and shock. *Orthop Clin North Am* 9:611, 1978

3. Trump BF: The role of cellular membrane systems in shock. In *The Cell in Shock*. Kalamazoo, Mich: The Upjohn Company, 1974

4. Trump BF, Berezesky IK, Cowley RA: The cellular and subcellular characteristics of acute and chronic injury with emphasis on the role of calcium. In *Pathophysiology of Shock, Anoxia, and Ischemia* (Trump BF, Cowley RA, eds). Baltimore: Williams & Wilkins, 1982

2

ASSESSING THE PATIENT IN SHOCK

JUDITH K. BOBB, RN, BSN

When the microcirculatory and cellular dysfunction that goes with shock is understood, assessment of the patient becomes easier. You can then focus on those parameters that will be most useful to your diagnosis. The key will be to look for evidence of decreased organ perfusion. Of course, therapy for shock must be initiated quickly. Therefore you should be able to recognize the clinical picture without undue loss of time.

In order to direct your assessment, however, you must first develop an index of suspicion. That is, you should be alert to deviations from the normal and know when such deviations may point to shock, which does not occur randomly. Examination of the patient's history will help you decide whether a risk exists.

History

Conditions in which to suspect shock

Hemorrhage/hypovolemia. Statistically, the most frequent cause of shock is hemorrhage and/or hypovolemia; therefore, the possibility of these should be considered first. In many instances, the potential for loss of intravascular volume is readily apparent (Table 2-1).

Loss of sympathetic tone. Shock following loss of sympathetic tone is a complication of spinal cord injury. This absence of vasoconstrictive stimulus greatly increases the vascular capacity, and the additional space cannot be filled by the normal blood volume. The result is likely to be decreased perfusion. In most individuals, vascular tone returns to normal in 3 to 4 days. In the interim, fluid support generally suffices to make up the relative deficit. The same is true for patients receiving spinal anesthesia. Care must be taken in both instances to avoid fluid overload once tonus is recovered.

Myocardial infarction. The combination of impaired left ventricular function and reduced total fluid intake

Table 2-1. Clinical Characteristics of Shock

1. Early shock	Increased sympathetic discharge	Normal BP, tachycardia Tachypnea, hyperpnea Alertness, good orientation, apprehension Pupils dilated Sweating
2. Middle shock	Decreased organ perfusion	BP normal or slightly decreased Disorientation, lethargy Decreased urine output Skin cool, moist
3. Late shock	Failure of compensation	Hypotension Lethargy Pulses weak Absent urine output Skin cold
4. Fourth-stage shock	Multiple organ failure	Loss of function in Lungs Kidneys Liver Cardiovascular instability Loss of host defenses Coagulopathy

poses the risk of increased interstitial fluid loss. Patients with impaired myocardial contractility or structural defects of the heart, as well as those receiving beta blockers, are also at risk for shock. Reduced cardiac output is also associated with cardiac arrhythmias (AV block, tachyarrhythmias, electromechanical dissociation) even if contractility is initially normal. In addition, there is evidence suggesting that repeated episodes of treatable shock will eventually lead to irreversible shock.

Sepsis. Sepsis often leads to shock. Of the estimated 330,000 annual cases of sepsis, approximately 40% progress to shock.[1] Although it is caused mainly by gram-negative organisms, sepsis has also been associated with gram-positive bacteria as well as viruses, rickettsiae, and fungi.[2] In toxic shock syndrome, described only recently, one of the diagnostic criteria is the presence of *Staphylococcus aureus.*[3]

Adrenal insufficiency. An unusual circumstance, one rarely mentioned in the literature, occurs when an individual with adrenal insufficiency suffers a shock-producing insult. Since these people cannot secrete enough norepinephrine (NE) and epinephrine (EPI) to maintain vascular tone, they are unlikely to survive without support from exogenous glucocorticoids. Clinically, their condition resembles neurogenic shock.

Inaccurate intake/output records. A recent study demonstrated a poor correlation between recorded totals and actual water balance.[4] By looking closely at patients as well as their records, the careful nurse can minimize the dangers of inadequate perfusion due to insufficient hydration.

Diagnostic tests with contrast media. Some contrast media—eg, barium—tend to produce osmotic water loss. Since patients undergoing diagnostic workups usually have been instructed to limit their oral fluid intake, they are likely to develop a degree of hypovolemia. After that, any additional loss of fluid volume, even if minor, can tip them into shock.

Shock of unexplained origin

The history serves to develop an index of suspicion where there is altered function. However, shock may also appear unannounced. Physical examination will then help to determine its cause. Since we cannot yet measure cell function directly, we must, instead, examine the function of critical organ systems.

Logic might suggest beginning with the cardiovascular system, since it is responsible for perfusion. However, the normal compensatory responses of the body frequently mask the cardiovascular signs of shock for some time. Therefore, you must look to the entire body's response as the basis for assessment, watching for both increased sympathetic discharge and decreased perfusion.

Clinical stages of shock

Shock may be delineated in terms of three main clinical stages:[5,6] (1) an early stage characterized by a generalized sympathetic nervous system response, (2) a middle stage revealing evidence of decreased tissue perfusion, and (3) a late stage marked by failure of compensatory responses. Successful resuscitation may still be accomplished at this last stage, although little time remains. Some patients who initially respond to therapy later lapse into a fourth stage, that of multiple organ failure (Table 2-1).

Early shock

Although shock begins with the onset of ischemia, this can generally be assumed to coincide with the moment of insult. During the ensuing hour, while most cells remain viable, the body mobilizes its resources in an attempt to correct the problem. During this phase, there is a marked increase in discharge by the sympathetic nervous system. Again, no single assessment parameter can support the diagnosis of shock; it is the *pattern* of the body's responses that must be observed.

This "fight or flight" reaction was first described by the noted physiologist Walter Cannon in the 1930s. When shock is the prime stimulus, only the degree and duration of activity differ from normal. In addition to direct action on many target organs, the release of NE from sympathetic nerve endings stimulates the release of more NE and EPI from the adrenal medulla. These two catecholamines increase the cardiac rate as well as

Table 2-2. Percentage of Blood in Vascular Compartments[7]

Heart	12	Arterioles	1
Lungs	18	Capillaries	5
Aorta	2	Venules, veins, and vena cava	54
Arteries	8		

the contractility of cardiac muscle. Arterioles in the skin, the gut, and the kidney become constricted. A physiologic diversion of blood from the venous capacitance to the arterial resistance side of the systemic circulation maintains blood pressure at or close to normal values (see Table 2-2).

In the lungs, EPI relaxes bronchial smooth muscle and increases the rate and depth of respiration. The threshold of the reticular activating system of the brain stem and spinal cord is lowered, producing an aroused, alert state. Apprehension and restlessness are also characteristic at this stage.

The muscles of the gut and bladder wall relax, while the bladder sphincter contracts. Contraction of the pilomotor and ciliary muscles produces gooseflesh and pupillary dilation. The sweat glands are also stimulated.

Invasive measurements of blood pressure (arterial, central venous, or pulmonary artery pressure) seldom provide diagnostic information at this stage, since these pressures are likely to be normal. The exception is when increased left ventricular end-diastolic pressure is reflected backward into the lungs and right atrium. Since this usually occurs in cardiogenic shock, it serves to support other clinical evidence but has little diagnostic value in itself.

Middle shock

As the effective cardiac output continues to fall, the patient passes into the middle phase of shock. Diminished

Table 2-3. Typical Arterial Blood Gases: Values in Hemorrhagic Shock and Normal Values

	SHOCK	NORMAL
Pa_{O2}	64 mm Hg	80 - 100 mm Hg
Pa_{CO2}	32 mm Hg	37 - 41 mm Hg
pH	7.47	7.35 - 7.45
HCO_3^-	20 mEq/L	21 - 27 mEq/L

organ perfusion becomes apparent. Diversion of blood from the skin and gut, increased vascular tone, and tachycardia tend to support the blood pressure. It falls, however, when 25 to 30% of the effective cardiac output is lost. The skin now becomes cool and pale.

An exception to this occurs in septic shock, where, it is believed, a decrease in peripheral vascular resistance leads to a maldistribution of the blood volume. Hence the so-called "warm shock," with warm, flushed skin.

Measurement of the blood pressure by sphygmomanometer is notoriously inaccurate at this stage; therefore measurement via an intraarterial line is essential. Since the amount of blood that can be diverted from the venous circulation is enormous, observed arterial pressures can also be nearly normal (Table 2-3). Except

Table 2-4. Invasive Vascular Pressures During Shock (Middle and Late)

	HYPOVOLEMIC	SEPTIC	CARDIOGENIC
Arterial BP	N to L	N	N to L
CVP	L	N to L	Elevated
PAP	L	N to L	Elevated

N = normal; L = low

when cardiac function is deranged, the CVP and PA pressures generally are low at this stage (Table 2-4).

The most significant finding during middle shock is the absence of adequate urinary output. Elevation of the circulating catecholamines, combined with a reduced cardiac output, is enough to cut off renal blood flow almost entirely. Additional causes of reduced urine flow include aldosterone-mediated sodium retention and water conservation produced by antidiuretic hormone. Both these hormones are liberated by sympathetic stimulation.

Late shock

Late shock coincides with transition to the point of no return. It is also the stage in septic shock when peripheral vascular resistance increases. Frank hypotension is present. The blood pressure may no longer be audible and the palpable pulse is difficult to locate, having often been described as weak and thready, with diminished amplitude. The patient may be unresponsive to all but noxious stimuli. The skin is cold and sometimes clammy, with an ashen, blue-gray appearance. Respirations continue to be rapid. Urine output is absent.

During this stage it may still be possible to resuscitate the patient through aggressive measures. If these fail, death must inevitably follow.

Multiple organ failure

Some patients who are successfully resuscitated ultimately decline into this fourth stage of shock. After several days of apparently normal recovery, such patients develop fever, cardiac instability, respiratory deterioration, and signs of sepsis. Initial success with cardiopulmonary support is followed by failure. Hepatic function deteriorates and renal failure ensues. Death is often marked by coagulopathy. Autopsy findings in the lungs are consistent with adult respiratory distress syndrome.

It has been suggested that the defect responsible for this syndrome involves the mitochondria, which are unable to utilize substrate for the generation of ATP.[8] Also implicated in this condition, as well as in septic shock, is the activation of complement, increased synthesis of prostaglandins and thromboxanes, and initiation of the coagulation cascade (see Chapter 9). The specific etiology remains to be discovered.

Laboratory assessment

Although there are no definitive laboratory tests for shock, several can help to gauge the syndrome's impact on the patient and may also serve to support the clinical findings.

Arterial blood gases

Arterial blood gases provide valuable information about the status of oxygenation and acid-base balance. An initial finding of hypoxemia supports the diagnosis of shock if no other cause is present (eg, preexisting disease, aspiration, chest injury). Reduced blood flow through the lungs impairs oxygen diffusion but has little effect on carbon dioxide removal. In fact, the usual response of the lungs is to increase carbon dioxide extraction, which is shown by a decrease in plasma CO_2 levels (Table 2-3).

It is commonly presumed that patients in shock will show metabolic acidosis, and tissue pH does fall during shock. However, though perfusion in the microcirculation is diminished, this will not show up as acidemia until the late stage.[9] Much more commonly, hyperventilation adequately maintains a normal pH or actually leads to respiratory alkalosis.

Glucose

Moderate hyperglycemia—due to epinephrine-induced glycogenolysis—is common. Insulin levels do not rise quickly, since EPI suppresses them and there is pancreatic hypoperfusion. In septic shock, insulin "resistance" may occur, impairing the hormone's ability to transport glucose across cell membranes.

Lactate

Anaerobic metabolic pathways increase the synthesis of lactate in the glycolytic cycle. The elevated serum lactate levels that result contribute to acidosis. Arterial lactate levels in excess of 15 mg/dL may show correlation with mortality and can therefore be useful predictors.

Osmolality, hematocrit

Contraction of the intravascular compartment due to hypovolemia may be reflected by an increase in plasma osmolality and hematocrit. Assessment of hematocrit in hemorrhagic shock has little initial value, since the losses are isotonic. Osmolality can be calculated if it is not available from the laboratory (Table 2-5).

Electrolytes

Shock rarely produces significant abnormalities of serum electrolytes. However, the underlying process may contribute to such abnormalities. Serum sodium and plasma osmolality reflect the status of fluid balance. Elevations in sodium reflect a relative water deficit.

Table 2-5. Calculation of Serum Osmolality from Serum Electrolytes

$$P_{osm} = (Na^{+} \times 2) + \frac{glucose}{18} + \frac{BUN}{2.8}$$

Note: Osmolality may be elevated by large molecules that are present but not usually measured (eg, alcohol, mannitol).

Baseline potassium measurements may uncover hypokalemia as a contributing factor in the development of shock. Good renal clearance of potassium by the normal kidney occurs despite major tissue injury. In fact, elevation of potassium should suggest acute renal impairment or failure as a complication.

Coagulation profile

Coagulopathy may complicate shock of any etiology. Defects are most often seen in septic and hemorrhagic shock. In many cases, they are revealed only by laboratory testing. Measurement of the prothrombin time, partial thromboplastin time, and platelet counts will reveal most current defects while also serving as a baseline for future comparison.

Urinalysis

After the patient has been catheterized and any residual urine has been discarded, a sample should be obtained for the measurement of urine sodium, osmolality, and creatinine (see Tables 10-1 and 10-2). The results help to distinguish oliguria due to hypovolemia from that of renal failure.

REFERENCES

1. Landesman SH, Gorbach SL: Gram negative sepsis and shock. *Orthop Clin North Am* 9:611, 1978

2. Weil MH, Shubin H: Bacterial shock. *JAMA* 235:421, 1976

3. Tofte RW, Williams DN: Toxic shock syndrome: Clinical and laboratory features in 15 patients. *Ann Intern Med* 94:149, 1981

4. Pflaum S: Investigation of intake-output as a means of assessing body fluid balance. *Heart Lung* 8:495, 1979

5. Trump BF: The role of cellular membrane systems in shock. In *The Cell in Shock*. Kalamazoo, Mich: The Upjohn Company, 1974

6. Trump BF, Berezesky IK, Cowley RA: The cellular and subcellular characteristics of acute and chronic injury with emphasis on the role of calcium. In *Pathophysiology of Shock, Anoxia, and Ischemia* (Trump BF, Cowley RA, eds). Baltimore: Williams & Wilkins, 1982

7. Gregg DE: Functional characteristics of the systemic and pulmonary circulation. In *The Physiological Basis of Medical Practice* (Best CH, Taylor NB, eds), 8th ed. Baltimore: Williams & Wilkins, 1966

8. Cerra FB, Border JR, McMenamy RH, Siegel JH: Multiple system organ failure. In *Pathophysiology of Shock, Anoxia, and Ischemia*. (Trump BF, Cowley RA, eds). Baltimore: Williams & Wilkins 1982

9. Wilson RF, Wilson JA, Gibson D, Sibbald WJ: Shock in the emergency department. *JACEP* 5:678, 1976

3

MONITORING THE PATIENT IN SHOCK

CLAREEN A. WIENCEK, RN, MSN, CCRN

Shock is characterized by inadequate tissue perfusion that can lead to organ or system failure; its nature and mechanisms are discussed in Chapter 1. Thorough, accurate, and continuous physiologic monitoring is essential both as a guide to therapy and to prevent the progression of shock.

With shock patients, commonly monitored parameters (eg, heart rate, respirations, temperature, and central venous pressure) are not always reliable indices of perfusion, tissue oxygenation, or patient survival.[1] Monitoring specific parameters of cardiorespiratory function and oxygen transport provides a better assessment of oxygen delivery and tissue perfusion.[2] The nurse plays a vital role in this process.

The care of shock patients, who are among the most acutely ill of those in the critical care setting, presents a unique challenge. The critical care nurse must not only excel in assessment and decision making but also understand the sophisticated equipment and techniques involved in monitoring the patient's hemodynamic status. These data must be gathered continuously, integrated with the underlying pathophysiology, and interpreted so as to guide nursing care.

Noninvasive monitoring

Physical assessment augments data provided by the more sophisticated invasive monitoring techniques, to be discussed later in this chapter. Although all body systems are included in the physical assessment of the patient in shock, the respiratory and cardiovascular systems are highlighted here.

Respiratory assessment

The first step in this assessment is to look at the patient's general work of breathing, noting bilateral chest expansion, use of accessory muscles, and skin color. Acid-base imbalances must be guarded against through scrutiny of arterial blood gases. If the patient is on a mechanical ventilator or has moderate to severe hypoxemia, respiratory alkalosis can occur. Accumulation of lactic acid in body tissues leads to metabolic acidosis. You must identify the type and cause of acid-base imbalance so that appropriate interventions can be instituted rapidly.

In auscultating the patient's lungs, you'll listen for pulmonary congestion by assessing the quality and location of adventitious breath sounds. (Such congestion is not expected in hypovolemic shock and septic shock but is usually associated with cardiogenic shock.)

Cardiovascular assessment

The anterior chest is inspected and palpated to provide information about the patient's cardiac status; then heart sounds are auscultated and correlated with the findings from inspection and palpation. The presence of S_3 gallop indicates left ventricular failure. The extremities are assessed to gather information about heart rate and stroke volume, both of which are affected in shock.

In the monitoring of arterial pulses, their presence, quality, and symmetry are noted. A weak or diminished pulse is expected in shock, but complete absence of the pulse is not; it may indicate systemic embolus, diffuse atherosclerosis, local thrombosis, or a dissecting aortic aneurysm. If the pulse diminishes significantly during inspiration and reappears during expiration, the patient may have pulsus paradoxus. Pulsus paradoxus would also be suggested by a decline of more than 10 mm Hg in the systolic blood pressure during inspiration, reflecting severe cardiac decompensation or tamponade. Severe left ventricular failure, in cardiogenic shock, may be associated with pulsus alternans. In this case, the pulse varies in amplitude from beat to beat.

The temperature of the extremities reflects the degree of peripheral vasoconstriction, a compensatory mechanism manifested by cool, clammy skin and weak pulses. The vasopressors often used to support blood pressure augment this effect. In the early stages of septic shock, however, the extremities may be flushed and warm because of increased metabolism, the febrile state, and regional venous pooling.

The extremities and nail beds are monitored for cyanosis, which becomes apparent peripherally when the arterial oxygen saturation is less than 75% (normal, 96 to 100%). Although the presence of cyanosis indicates tissue hypoxia, its absence does not confirm adequate perfusion and oxygenation.[3]

Invasive monitoring

Components of the pressure-monitoring system

A fluid-filled system is used to monitor arterial and other internal pressures directly. A balloon-tipped catheter is inserted through a peripheral vein or percutaneously into the patient's right atrium and ventricle and then into the pulmonary artery. This catheter, made of polyvinyl tubing, runs to a pressure transducer, which converts the mechanical energy transmitted by the catheter into electrical impulses. These impulses are amplified and displayed as a waveform on an oscilloscope. A correctly placed catheter, fluid-filled system (no air bubbles), and reliable transducer are essential to accurate pressure monitoring. No matter what pressure is being measured, the components of the system are basically the same (Figure 3-1).

In addition to the oscilloscope, a strip-chart recorder may be used to obtain a permanent record of pressure values. When a recorder with two or more channels is used, the ECG and up to three pressures can be ob-

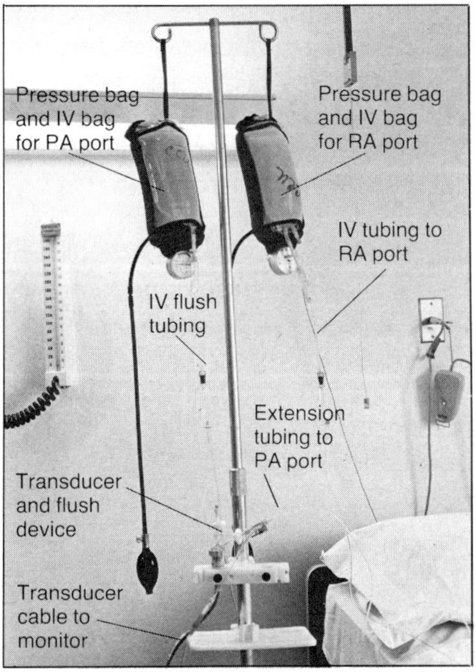

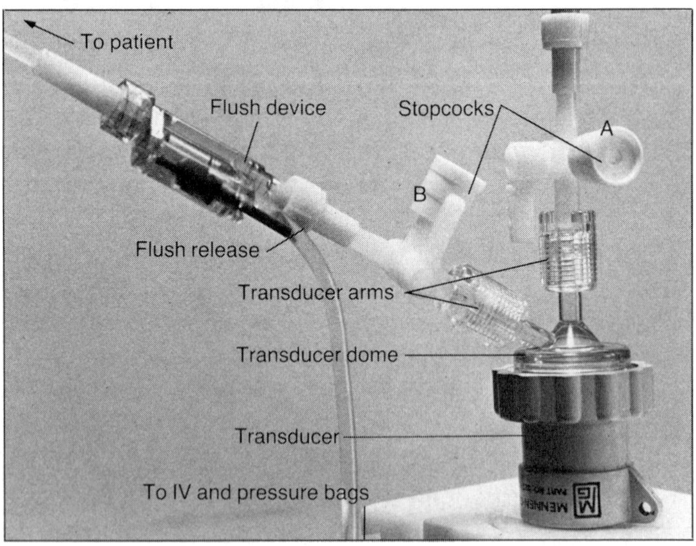

Figure 3-1. Two views of an arterial pressure-monitoring system.

tained simultaneously. This makes it possible to analyze the mechanical components of the pressure waveform in relation to the electrical events of the ECG, and thus to interpret pressure readings more accurately.

All systems require zero balancing—negating the effects of atmospheric pressure—and calibration before pressures can be relied on as accurate.

Invasive monitoring of directly measured parameters

The cardiorespiratory and oxygen transport variables are either measured directly or derived from one or more directly obtained values. The remainder of this chapter will focus on the definition and significance of these parameters, on monitoring techniques, and on expected variations in shock states. The directly measured indicators of cardiovascular function include:

1. Mean arterial pressure
2. Pulmonary artery pressure
3. Pulmonary artery wedge pressure, or pulmonary capillary wedge pressure
4. Central venous pressure
5. Cardiac output.

Mean arterial pressure

Arterial blood pressure reflects the volume and flow of blood in the vascular system. The standard method of measuring this pressure, with arm cuff and sphygmomanometer, suffices for the stable patient. Arm cuff pressures are not entirely accurate, however, usually varying up to 10% from directly monitored arterial pressure.[4] Moreover, the shock syndrome is usually associated with compensatory peripheral vasoconstriction and often with low cardiac output. Both conditions make measurement of blood pressure with an arm cuff difficult because of diminished or absent Korotkoff's sounds. Therefore, intraarterial pressure lines should be inserted so that blood pressure monitoring is continuous and accurate.

Physiologic components of blood pressure. The arterial blood pressure is composed of systole and diastole; pulse pressure is the difference between the systolic value and the diastolic value. Normal systolic arterial pressure is 100 to 140 mm Hg. It reflects the degree of systemic vascular resistance and compliance of the arteries. The normal diastolic pressure is 60 to 90 mm Hg and reflects the velocity of runoff of blood from the aorta, the elasticity of the arterial walls, and the degree of vasoconstriction.

In evaluating the intraarterial pressure of the patient in shock, the mean arterial pressure (MAP) must be monitored. The MAP is the average pressure pushing blood through the systemic circulation, ensuring tissue blood flow. Since the common denominator in shock is inadequate tissue perfusion, the MAP reflects the degree of shock.

Pressure-regulatory mechanisms maintain the MAP within narrow limits of 80 to 120 mm Hg, the average being 100 mm Hg. The MAP is not a true mean because diastole makes up more of the cardiac cycle than does systole. The following formula is used to calculate the MAP:

$$\text{MAP} = \frac{\text{systolic pressure} + 2(\text{diastolic pressure})}{3}$$

The two major determinants of MAP are cardiac output (CO) and systemic vascular resistance (SVR). A change in CO or SVR would cause a change in the MAP. The body's regulatory mechanisms maintain the MAP within narrow limits by regulating either or both of these components. The regulatory mechanisms include neural, hormonal, and renal control mechanisms.

Neural mechanisms act through the baroreceptors and chemoreceptors to maintain MAP. They act rapidly to prevent minute-by-minute fluctuations in blood pressure due to exercise and changes in position and abdominal tone.

Hormonal regulatory mechanisms can also act rapidly to control MAP. These include direct sympathetic stimulation to peripheral vessels and indirect stimulation through the release of catecholamines.

Although the neural mechanism specifically and, to a lesser degree, the hormonal mechanism act rapidly to prevent fluctuations in MAP, they eventually lose their responsiveness and the ability to control MAP. For long-term pressure control, the renal body-fluid pressure-control system is activated.[4] Basically, this system maintains MAP through the retention of sodium and water, increasing blood volume and CO.

Blood pressure in shock. Hypotension is usually associated with the shock state, but the blood pressure may initially be normal or high because of compensatory mechanisms mediated by the sympathetic nervous system. The sympathetic reflexes increase the MAP more by increasing SVR than by increasing CO. With an increase in SVR, diastole increases and the pulse pressure narrows. Thus, the pulse pressure becomes significant as a measure of stroke volume and degree of vasoconstriction.

Though continuous monitoring of MAP will reflect the degree of shock, it does not bear a consistent relationship to total blood flow.[5] A patient in shock may have a normal blood pressure and cardiac output while perfusion is still inadequate to meet the tissue needs. Other parameters, described later, have been found to be better predictors of survival for the patient in shock.[1]

Techniques of intraarterial pressure monitoring. Intraarterial pressure is directly monitored through the insertion and maintenance of a flexible polyvinyl catheter, usually 5 to 6 cm long, into a readily accessible artery. The most common access sites for an arterial line include the radial, brachial, and femoral arteries. The radial artery is the preferred site because of easy accessibility, more effective stabilization once inserted, better control of bleeding around the insertion site, and usually good collateral circulation to the hand.

Prior to insertion of a radial arterial line, Allen's test should be performed to assess adequacy of collateral circulation. To perform this test, occlude the radial and ulnar arteries simultaneously with firm digital pressure until blanching is observed. If blood supply to the hand through the ulnar artery is adequate, the hand will quickly change from blanched to pink after the ulnar artery is released while the radial artery is still occluded.

The normal arterial presure waveform (Figure 3-2) obtained through invasive monitoring has a distinct appearance, being composed of a rapid systolic upstroke, clear dicrotic notch, and diastole. The dicrotic notch, located on the downstroke, represents a temporary increase in aortic pressure when the aortic valve closes. End diastole is the lowest pressure point just prior to the next systole. If the systolic upstroke is slow and rounded and the dicrotic notch is poorly defined, the pressure waveform is described as damped (Figure 3-3). This can indicate a clot in the catheter, loss of pressure in the

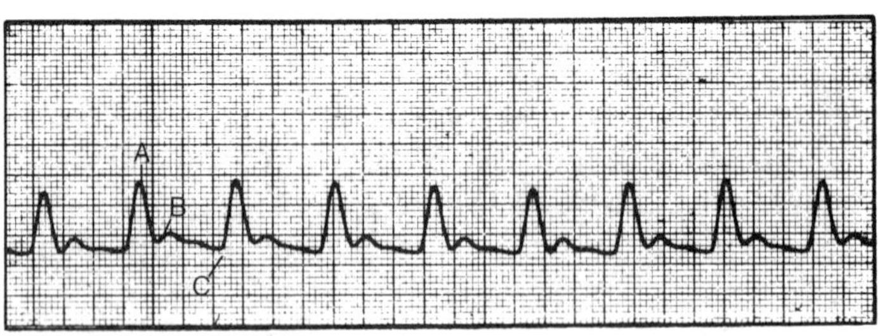

Figure 3-2. Normal arterial pressure waveform. A = rapid systolic upstroke; B = dicrotic notch; C = end-diastole.

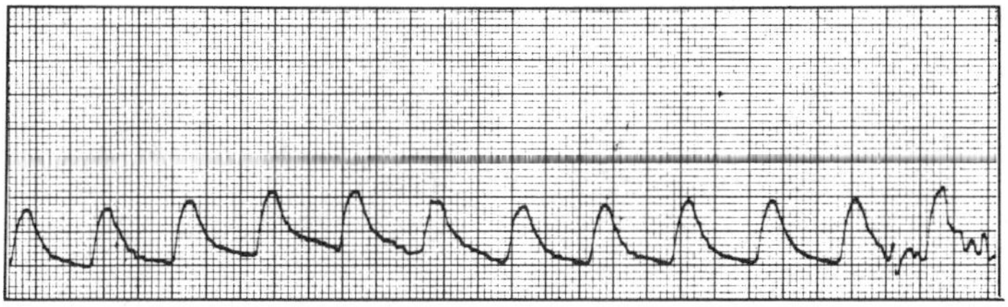

Figure 3-3. Damped arterial pressure waveform. Note the loss of rapid systolic upstroke and dicrotic notch.

system, air in the line, or pressure of the catheter tip against the vessel wall. You must be able to distinguish a damped waveform due to these causes from a waveform due to low MAP.

The nurse plays a central role in intraarterial pressure monitoring. Once the arterial catheter is inserted and secured, it is the nurse who collects ongoing data about the patient's blood pressure. The following measures will ensure the patient's safety and elicit the most accurate and reliable data from arterial lines:

1. Monitoring alarms should be on at all times to alert the nurse to disconnection or a drop or increase in pressure.
2. The circulation, pulses, color, temperature, and movement of the extremity distal to the insertion site should be monitored frequently.
3. The extremity should be immobilized with an arm board to minimize movement of the catheter in the vessel and irritation to the vessel wall.
4. The line should be removed after 72 to 96 hours to reduce the chance of infection.[3]
5. Periodically, check for adequate pressure in the pressure bag and tight connections so as to prevent blood backup and ensure proper functioning of the flush device.
6. Low blood pressure and low flow states, as seen in shock, may require fast flushing on a regular basis to maintain patency of the catheter; frequently as-

sess the quality of the pressure waveform as an index of clot formation and catheter patency.

Pulmonary artery pressure

Floating balloon catheters. Hemodynamic monitoring with floating balloon catheters (Swan-Ganz type) has come into widespread use for the care of patients in shock. These are balloon-tipped, flow-directed catheters inserted through right heart catheterization into the pulmonary artery. They make possible the direct measurement of right atrial (RA) pressure, pulmonary artery (PA) pressure, pulmonary artery wedge (PAW) pressure, cardiac output, and mixed venous gases. These parameters provide valuable information about the fluid and cardiac status of the patient in shock, about left ventricular function, and about the patient's response to therapy.

The pulmonary artery catheter (Figure 3-4) is a flexible catheter made of polyvinyl chloride; it is 110 cm long and marked in 10-cm increments. At present, there are two-, three, four-, and the newly developed five-lumen catheters.

Each lumen has a specific function. The proximal, or central venous pressure (CVP), lumen is used as a central line for fluid administration or as a pressure-monitoring line to record RA pressure. The opening of the proximal lumen is located 30 cm from the tip and sits in or near the right atrium. The opening of the distal lumen is located at the tip of the catheter and sits in the PA. PA pressures, PAW pressures, and mixed venous gases are obtained through this port. The thermistor lumen contains temperature-sensitive wires for determining CO by the thermodilution technique. The thermistor bead, or end of this lumen, is found 4 cm from the catheter tip, located in the PA. The fourth lumen is for inflation and deflation of the thin latex balloon that surrounds, but does not cover, the tip of the catheter when inflated. All pulmonary artery catheters have at least the distal lumen and the balloon-inflation lumen.

The catheter can be inserted at the bedside. Fluoroscopy is not required for insertion because of the characteristic pressures obtained in each chamber. However, some physicians choose to use fluoroscopy as an additional guide during insertion. The catheter can be insert-

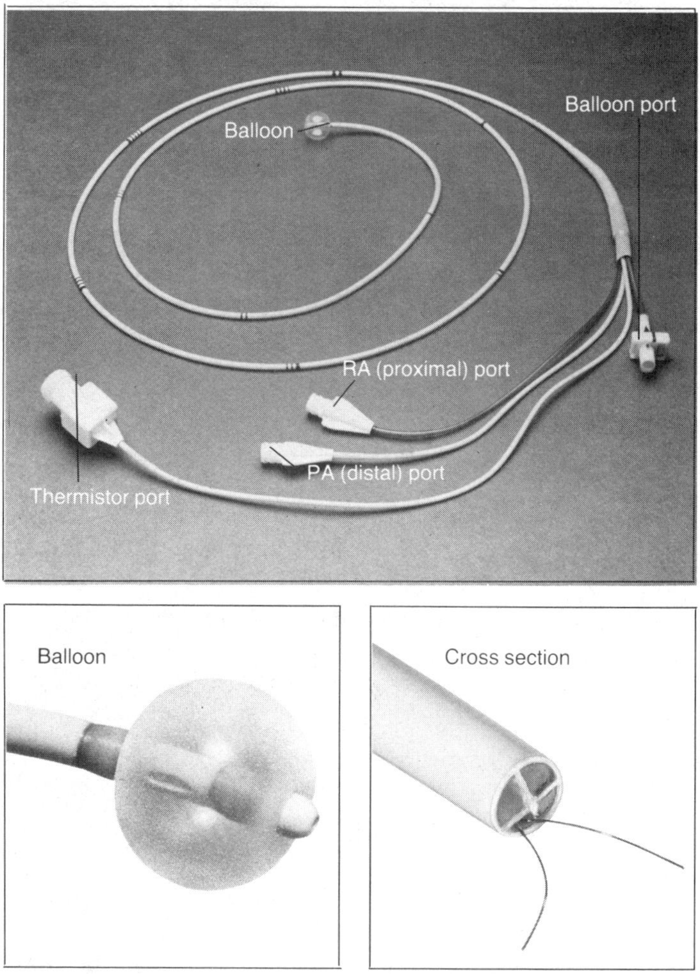

Figure 3-4. The four-lumen thermodilution floating balloon catheter.

ed via a peripheral or central vein, either percutaneously or via cutdown. Potential sites include the subclavian, internal jugular, basilic, and cephalic veins.

Significance and waveform analysis. PA pressures, continuously monitored through the distal lumen of the catheter, give an estimate of the venous pressure within the lungs. Normal PA pressures range from 20 to 30 mm Hg systolic, and from 10 to 20 mm Hg diastolic; the mean PA pressure is 10 to 15 mm Hg.

Continuous PAP monitoring is important for several reasons:

1. Therapy depends on these measurements.
2. It detects changes in the position of the catheter tip.
3. It can help prevent pulmonary infarction, which may occur when the catheter spontaneously moves to the wedge position with the balloon deflated—usually, but not always, within a few hours after insertion.[6]

The PA pressure waveform has a definite, rapid systolic upstroke due to right ventricular ejection, a dicrotic notch caused by closure of the pulmonic valve, and end diastole. The PA end-diastolic pressure is the lowest pressure point just prior to the next systole. If the PA pressure fluctuates significantly with respirations, it should be read at the end-expiration point.[7]

PA pressures will be increased by pulmonary hypertension, pulmonary embolus, high levels of positive end-expiratory pressure (PEEP), and pulmonary congestion secondary to left ventricular failure. Assuming there is no related lung pathology, expect the PA pressure to be increased in cardiogenic shock, but to be normal or decreased in septic and hypovolemic shock.

Pulmonary artery wedge pressure

As the balloon of the pulmonary artery catheter is inflated, the tip becomes buoyant and is carried in the direc-

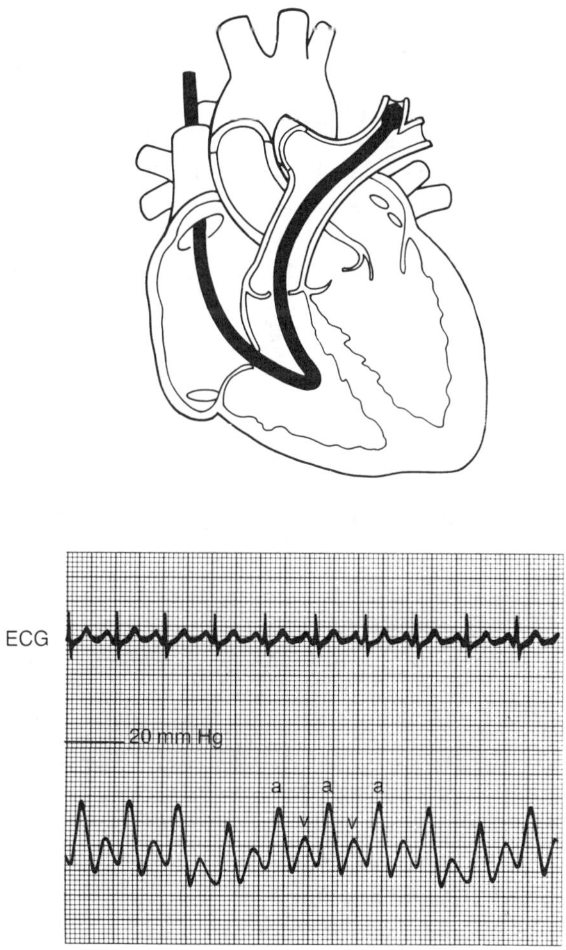

Figure 3-5. The catheter in the wedged position, with a typical PAW pressure tracing. The a waves and v waves are present; the c waves are not. ECG and PAW pressure tracings reproduced, with permission, from Hudak CM, Lohr T, Gallo BM: Critical Care Nursing, 3rd ed. Philadelphia: Lippincott, 1982.

tion of blood flow to a smaller branch of the pulmonary arterial tree. When the diameter of the balloon is the same as or less than the vessel diameter, the catheter wedges in the vessel. At this point, there is no blood flow past the inflated balloon and the tip of the catheter "views" the more distal pulmonary capillary system. In the wedged position, the distal lumen is no longer sensing PA pressures, but rather the pressure transmitted back through the pulmonary vascular bed from the left side of the heart. More specifically, the pulmonary artery wedge (PAW) directly reflects the left atrial (LA) pressure and left ventricular end-diastolic pressure (LVEDP). At end diastole, when the mitral valve is still open, these pressures are equilibrated and transmitted back through the pulmonary vasculature to the catheter tip in the wedged position.

Monitoring of LVEDP through the PAW pressure is the method used for clinical assessment of LV preload, a major determinant of LV function. Starling's law of the heart states that the greater the diastolic volume in the ventricle, the more the fibers are stretched and the more forceful the subsequent contraction. In most situations, increasing the LV preload will increase the force of contraction and the stroke volume (SV). An increase in preload does not always improve ventricular contraction, however. If the ventricle becomes overloaded, as in congestive heart failure (CHF) or cardiogenic shock, a further increase in the diastolic volume or preload can impair LV function significantly.

The PAW pressure is also an index of pulmonary congestion. Since the pulmonary capillary pressure is a major determinant of fluid movement between the vascular bed and the interstitial spaces and alveoli, the higher the wedge pressure, the more fluid that escapes into the interstitial tissues. The primary cause of high pulmonary artery wedge pressures and pulmonary congestion is a failing left ventricle.

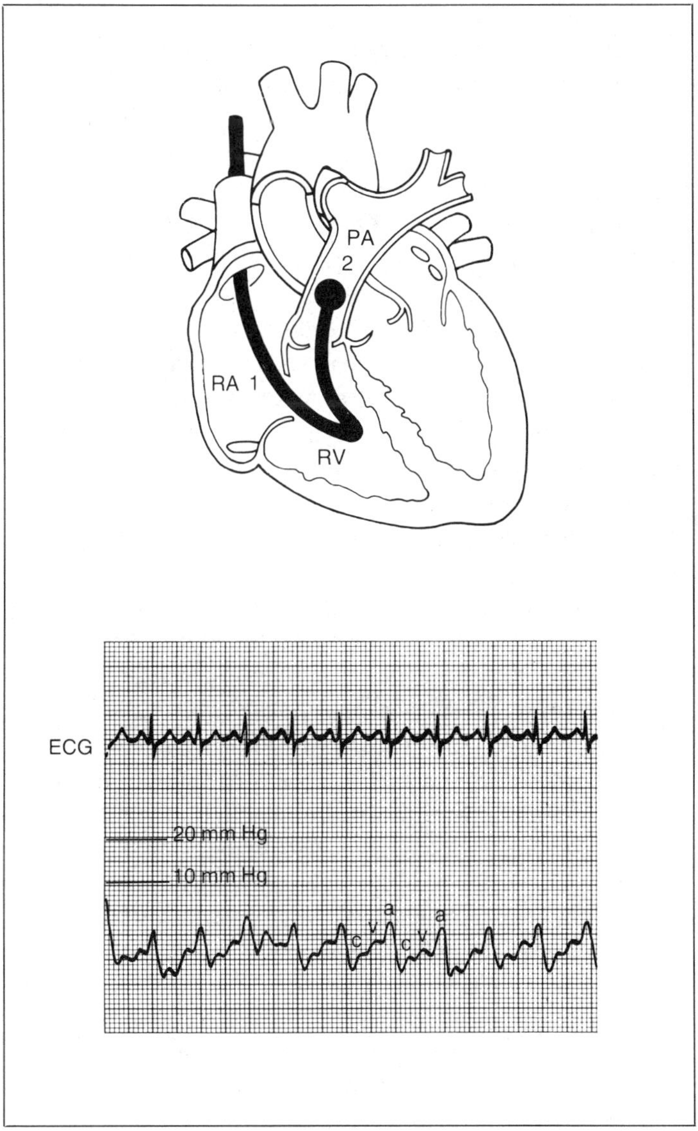

Figure 3-6. RA pressure tracing obtained via the proximal lumen of the catheter. 1 = proximal port; 2 = distal port. ECG and RA pressure tracings reproduced, with permission, from Hudak CM, Lohr T, Gallo BM: Critical Care Nursing, 3rd ed. Philadelphia: Lippincott, 1982

There are some limitations to the use of the PAW pressure as an index of LVEDP. In the presence of mitral valve insufficiency, the mean PAW pressure is not a reliable indicator of LVEDP. In these cases, the mean PAW pressure is elevated and the *a* wave of the PAW tracing more accurately reflects the LVEDP.[3]

In addition to the PAW pressure, the PA end-diastolic pressure can be used to assess LVEDP. The PA end-diastolic pressure and the PAW pressure normally do not vary by more than a few millimeters of mercury; these pressures are nearly the same when pulmonary vascular resistance is normal.[3] Because there is risk of pulmonary infarction when wedging the catheter and the catheter at times cannot be wedged, the PA end-diastolic pressure can be used to determine the LVEDP. However, certain pathologic states such as pulmonary hypertension, chronic obstructive pulmonary disease, pulmonary embolus, and hypoxia will increase the PA pressure while the PAW pressure may remain normal. The presence of these pathologies necessitates direct measurement of the PAW pressure as an index of LVEDP.[3]

Measuring PAW pressures. The normal PAW pressure is a mean pressure of 4 to 12 mm Hg. Its waveform (Figure 3-5) has three components. The *a* wave is produced by LA systole and falls slightly after the P wave of the ECG. The *c* wave, often not seen in the tracing, represents closure of the mitral valve at the beginning of ventricular systole. The *v* wave reflects bulging of the mitral valve back into the LA during LV systole. It follows the T wave of the ECG. As with PA pressures, PAW pressures may also fluctuate with the respiratory cycle (increased with expiration, decreased with inspiration) and should be measured at the end-expiration point.

When monitoring the patient in shock, measure PA pressures continuously and obtain PAW pressures approximately every 2 to 4 hours. The condition of some patients may require more frequent wedge pressures, but this is not recommended because it risks pulmonary infarction and balloon rupture. The steps for obtaining a wedge pressure are as follows:

1. Place the patient in the flat, supine position.
2. Position the air-fluid interface of the transducer at the level of the RA (midaxillary line).
3. Zero balance the transducer.
4. Slowly inflate the balloon while continuously watching the pressure monitor; balloon capacity is 1.25 to 1.5 mL of air, but usually only 0.8 to 1.0 mL are required to wedge.
5. If you do not feel a slight resistance while inflating the balloon, it may be ruptured; discontinue the procedure.
6. Stop inflating the balloon as soon as the distal lumen waveform changes from a PA pressure waveform to a PAW pressure waveform.
7. Observe the monitor for a few seconds and record PAW pressure.
8. Detach the tuberculin syringe from the balloon inflation lumen and allow air to come out.
9. Verify that the catheter is no longer wedged by watching for the spontaneous return of the PA pressure waveform.

PAW pressures in shock. Hypovolemic, early septic, and neurogenic shock are usually associated with low wedge pressures.[6] Hypovolemic shock is due to a decrease in both circulating volume and venous return, which leads to lower filling pressures. Thus, low PAW pressures are expected in these patients. In early septic shock, low PAW pressure reflects relative hypovolemia secondary to diffuse vasodilation and fluid shifts from the vascular space. The PAW pressure is low in neurogenic shock because of the peripheral vasodilation and decreased venous return.

Cardiogenic shock is associated with high PAW pressures because of LV pump failure. The elevated wedge pressure indicates the LV's inability to handle its venous return, or preload. A wedge pressure above normal reflects dysfunction of the LV, whether mild, moderate, or severe. Pulmonary congestion usually begins with wedge pressures around 18 mm Hg; pressures greater than 25 mm Hg indicate impending or existing pulmonary edema.[3] These values, however, vary considerably from patient to patient. A PAW pressure of 18 mm Hg may signal pulmonary edema in one patient but may go as high as 28 mm Hg in another individual.

Central venous pressure

Central venous pressure (CVP) reflects the pressure in the RA. It is used to monitor blood volume and venous return to the right side of the heart. The CVP is a much less sensitive indicator of left heart function than the PAW pressure; thus, the latter is monitored predominantly in shock. Although the CVP tends to follow the wedge pressure, it is the last to change and is an inadequate guide to therapy in myocardial dysfunction, poor perfusion, sepsis, and severe hemorrhage.[2]

CVP or the RA pressure can be obtained by pressure monitoring via the proximal lumen of the pulmonary artery catheter. The transducer and pressure monitoring line are the same as for PA pressures. The RA pressure is normally 2 to 6 mm Hg (Figure 3-6).

A central line, inserted percutaneously or via a cutdown, and a water manometer can also be used to obtain the CVP—in this case, measured in centimeters of water, the normal range being 5 to 15 cm H_2O.

Invasive monitoring—derived calculations

Direct measurement of the intraarterial pressure via an arterial line and the PA and PAW pressure via the balloon-tipped, flow-directed catheter provide valuable data about the status of the patient in shock. Two additional parameters, cardiac output and mixed venous gases, can also be directly obtained with the catheter. These two parameters bear an integral relationship with derived parameters.

Once direct measurements are taken on the patient in shock, other parameters need to be assessed through derived calculations. A more complete picture of the patient's cardiorespiratory and oxygen transport status is gained when derived variables are monitored. These parameters include stroke index, cardiac index, systemic vascular resistance, left ventricular stroke work, the left ventricular function curve, and arteriovenous oxygen content difference. Direct measurement of the patient's serum lactate level completes the cardiovascular assessment.

Cardiac output and cardiac index

Appropriate care and treatment of the patient in shock require monitoring of the CO and the cardiac index (CI) as parameters of LV function. CO is the amount of blood pumped by the heart per minute, approximately 4 to 8 L/min. The CO determines the transport of blood, oxygen, and other essential nutrients to the tissues. Since the major physiologic defect in shock is inadequate perfusion, the CO provides essential information about the degree of shock, LV function, and overall cardiac status.

CO can be measured with a four-lumen thermodilution catheter. A parameter easily derived from the CO is the CI, a more specific measurement of LV function because it accounts for body size. CI is equal to the CO per square meter of body surface area (BSA):

$$CI = \frac{CO}{BSA\ (m^2)}$$

The patient's BSA can be obtained from standard charts when height and weight are known. The normal CI is 2.5 to 4 $L/min/m^2$.

Example: A 70-kg man is 6 ft tall. According to a standard BSA chart, he has a BSA of 1.9 m^2. His cardiac output is 6 L/min. Thus, the CI is 3.15 $L/min/m^2$.

CO is the product of heart rate and stroke volume. SV is the amount of blood pumped by the ventricle with each beat, approximately 60 to 130 mL. The stroke index (SI) can be calculated by dividing the CI (multiplied by 1,000 to convert liters to milliliters) by pulse rate. The normal SI is 35 to 70 $mL/beat/m^2$.

The major determinant of CO is venous return, the amount of blood returned to the heart from the peripheral circulation. Venous return is determined primarily by the degree of systemic vascular resistance (SVR), so that CO is regulated by changes in the SVR. The degree of vasodilation or vasoconstriction at the tissue level will affect the SVR. The greater the vasoconstriction, the greater the SVR and the greater the venous return. This ability of the tissues to control blood flow in accordance with their needs is called autoregulation. Many of the compensatory mechanisms associated with shock work by increasing the SVR and/or heart rate in an effort to increase or maintain the CO.

SVR can be monitored in the clinical setting as a derived calculation. It is calculated with this formula:

$$SVR = \frac{(MAP - CVP)79.9}{CO}$$

The normal SVR is 900 to 1,600 $dyne/sec/cm^5$. SVR is elevated in hypovolemic, late septic, and cardiogenic shock as a result of the compensatory vasoconstriction mediated by the sympathetic nervous system in an attempt to increase the venous return, the SV, and eventually the CO. The SVR is diminished in states of vasodilation such as early septic shock.

The heart itself plays a permissive role in CO regulation under normal conditions. The heart pumps whatever venous return it receives up to 13 to 15 L/min. Thus, venous return controls the CO whenever the permissive level of the heart is greater.[4] The heart becomes the limiting factor in CHF and LV failure.

Measurement of cardiac output. The most frequent method used to measure CO at the bedside is the thermodilution technique. This requires a four-lumen thermodilution pulmonary artery catheter and calculates CO based on temperature change. A 10-mL bolus of 5% dextrose in water or 0.9 N saline is injected through the proximal port into the RA. The injected fluid must be cooler than the patient's blood to effect a temperature change that will be sensed. The temperature change that occurs as the bolus mixes with the SV pumped out of the RV is "read" downstream by the thermistor bead in the PA. The signal is then transmitted back through the thermistor wires to the CO computer and displayed in liters per minute. (If fluids are restricted and only a 5-mL bolus is injected, adjust the "cal" factor on the CO machine.)

The thermodilution CO technique can be done easily and as often as necessary by the nurse monitoring the patient. It is relatively quick and safe for the patient. Iced or room-temperature fluid can be used, though iced fluid is used more frequently because it results in greater temperature change. The solution is injected quickly and steadily within 4 seconds. Usually, three CO measurements are made and then averaged. Once CO is obtained, the CI can be calculated.

Monitoring left ventricular performance in shock. As shock progresses, no matter what the initiating event, the heart begins to deteriorate, facilitating the progression. It is the deterioration of the heart itself, whether from poor perfusion or a myocardial toxic factor, that makes shock irreversible.[4]

Because myocardial function is a deciding factor in survival, monitoring of LV performance is essential. Three determinants of LV function—preload, afterload, and heart rate—can be monitored clinically. The fourth determinant—contractility—is more commonly inferred than directly measured. CO is the product of the effects of these four factors on ventricular function.

Preload, as described earlier, is the volume in the LV at the end of diastole. It is the filling pressure and determines the degree of fiber stretching. The greater the preload, the more forceful the contraction. Thus, in most circumstances, CO varies directly with preload. Preload is measured clinically as PAW pressure. Afterload is equivalent to the impedance or resistance to LV ejection; the greater the afterload, the harder the LV must work to eject its stroke volume. Therefore, LV output usually varies inversely with afterload. Systolic arterial pressure is used to monitor afterload. Heart rate also affects LV performance and CO. CO varies directly with heart rates of less than 160/min. Heart rates greater than 160/min do not allow for adequate diastolic filling; thus the SV decreases. The contractile state of the myocardial fibers is the final determinant of LV function. Intimately related to preload and afterload, contractility is also affected by sympathetic influences, drugs, and disease.

The CO will be decreased in cardiogenic shock because of the LV's impaired pumping ability. As the ventricle fails, the preload, or LVEDP, rises significantly above normal. As a compensatory mechanism for the shock syndrome, SVR increases, which in turn increases the afterload. Because it is harder for the LV to eject blood, residual volume or preload increases and further impairs LV function. A CI of less than 2.2 $L/min/m^2$ is used to differentiate cardiogenic shock from other types.

In hypovolemic shock, there is an absolute deficiency in blood volume, which leads to decreased venous return and preload. The result is a low PAW pressure and low CO. The SVR increases to compensate for the decrease in venous return; since myocardial function is generally normal, however, this increase in afterload does not increase the preload, as in cardiogenic shock.

The monitoring parameters in septic shock will vary depending on whether the patient is in the early or late stage. In early septic shock, the widespread vasodilation and regional pooling lead to a relative decrease in blood volume. The low venous return is reflected in low PA and PAW pressures. The low SVR plus compensatory mechanisms—such as tachycardia and greater myocardial contractility—facilitate LV ejection and the CO tends to be far above normal.

In late septic shock, vasoconstriction prevails but a volume deficit persists from trapping of blood in regional beds and leakage of plasma from the capillaries into the extravascular spaces. Cardiac function deteriorates and CO decreases because of the depression of myocardial contractility and the greater afterload, or SVR, which it cannot overcome.

Table 3-1. Expected Values of Hemodynamic Parameters in Different Types of Shock

	CO/CI	PAP	PAWP	SVR
Cardiogenic shock	↓	↑	↑	↑
Hypovolemic shock	↓	↓	↓	↑
Early septic shock	↑	↓	↓	↓
Late septic shock	↓	↓	↓	↑
Neurogenic shock	N or ↑	↓	↓	↓

Legend: ↑ = increased above normal value
↓ = decreased below normal value
N = normal

Neurogenic shock is caused by peripheral vasodilation secondary to loss of vasomotor tone. The decrease in both venous return and SVR is reflected in low PAW and PA pressures. The decrease in SVR facilitates LV ejection, so the CO may be normal or high if the patient's initial blood volume was adequate. Table 3-1 summarizes the expected values of CO, PA pressure, PAW pressure, and SVR in the different types of shock.

Contractility, preload, afterload, and heart rate must be considered in monitoring the CO and overall LV performance of the patient in shock. The parameters of myocardial function can be monitored separately in the clinical setting or collectively as they affect LV performance. The ventricular function curve (Figure 3-7) incorporates the four determinants and is one of the best ways to monitor the heart's functional ability.[2]

The ventricular function curve plots left ventricular stroke work (LVSW) against LVEDP or PAW pressure. LVSW quantitates the amount of work the LV does with each beat and is another way of evaluating the pumping ability of the ventricle. The normal LVSW is 45 to 85 gram-meters per square meter of body surface (g-m/m^2) and is calculated by using this formula:

$$\text{LVSW} = \frac{\text{CI(MAP} - \text{PAWP)13.6}}{\text{heart rate}}$$

The LVSW tends to be decreased in hypovolemic shock because of low circulatory volume. In cardiogenic shock, LVSW will be low because of the primary defect of impaired pumping ability. In septic shock, the LVSW may be low because of myocardial depressant factor or decreased coronary perfusion.

When the LVSW is plotted against the LVEDP, the factors affecting LV performance are integrated. The resulting value or point on the curve indicates the degree of myocardial contractility. The zone of normal ventricular function is indicated by the shaded area on the curve in Figure 3-7. If the single-point plot falls outside the shaded zone, the patient's myocardial performance is impaired.

Arteriovenous oxygen difference. Monitoring the arteriovenous oxygen difference (a-vDO_2) augments the assessment of respiratory and oxygen transport status in the shock patient. a-vDO_2 is the difference between the oxygen content in arterial blood and mixed

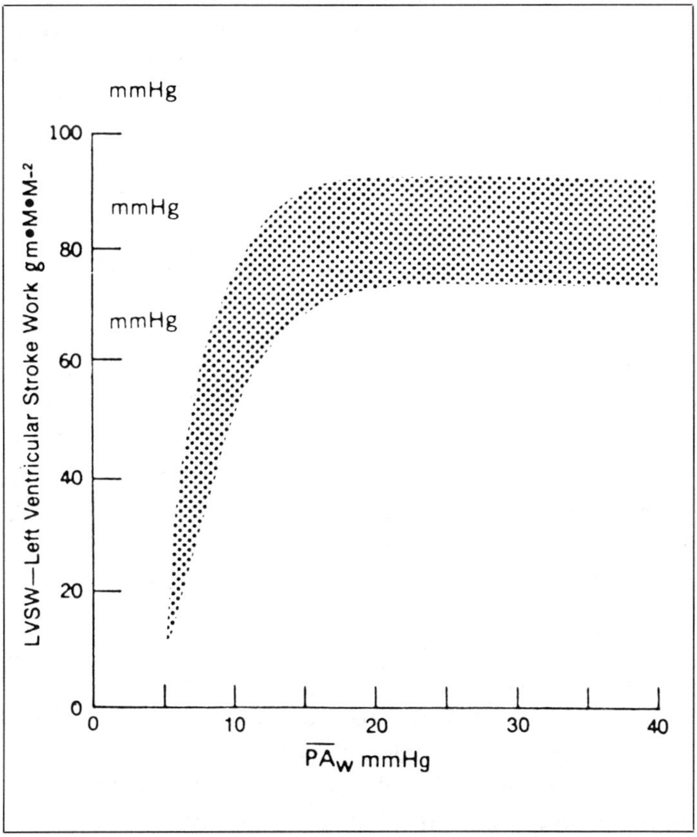

Figure 3-7. Ventricular function curve for a patient in septic shock. The shaded area is the range of normal ventricular function.

venous blood and measures the extent to which blood flow matches the metabolic demand for oxygen. The normal a-vDO_2 is 3.0 to 5.5 vol% (mL/100 mL).

The arterial oxygen content is derived from the arterial oxygen saturation (SaO_2) obtained from arterial blood gases. Mixed venous gases must be drawn to measure the venous oxygen saturation (SvO_2) and calculate the venous oxygen content. In the clinical setting, the distal lumen of the pulmonary artery catheter is used to obtain mixed venous gases from the PA. Since each gram of hemoglobin can carry 1.34 mL of oxygen when 100% saturated, the oxygen content is calculated using this formula:

$$\text{Arterial } O_2 \text{ content (vol\%)} = 1.34 \times \text{amount of Hb} \times SaO_2$$

$$\text{Venous } O_2 \text{ content (vol\%)} = 1.34 \times \text{amount of Hb} \times SvO_2$$

In the normal resting state, the tissues consume only 25% of the oxygen delivered by the CO. Because of this large oxygen reserve, the normal arterial O_2 saturation is 96 to 100% and the normal venous O_2 saturation is 75%. A venous O_2 saturation below normal indicates either that increased oxygen demands are not being met or that the amount of available oxygen is decreased. If less oxygen is available, the tissues extract more, resulting in a lower venous O_2 saturation. This will increase the a-vDO_2 above normal.

The a-vDO_2 varies inversely with the CO. When CO and blood flow to the tissues are decreased, the tissues compensate by extracting a higher proportion of oxygen, and therefore the blood returning to the heart will have a lower than normal oxygen content. Monitoring a-vDO_2 in the shock patient provides information about CO. An a-vDO_2 above 5.5 vol% indicates low cardiac output.[3]

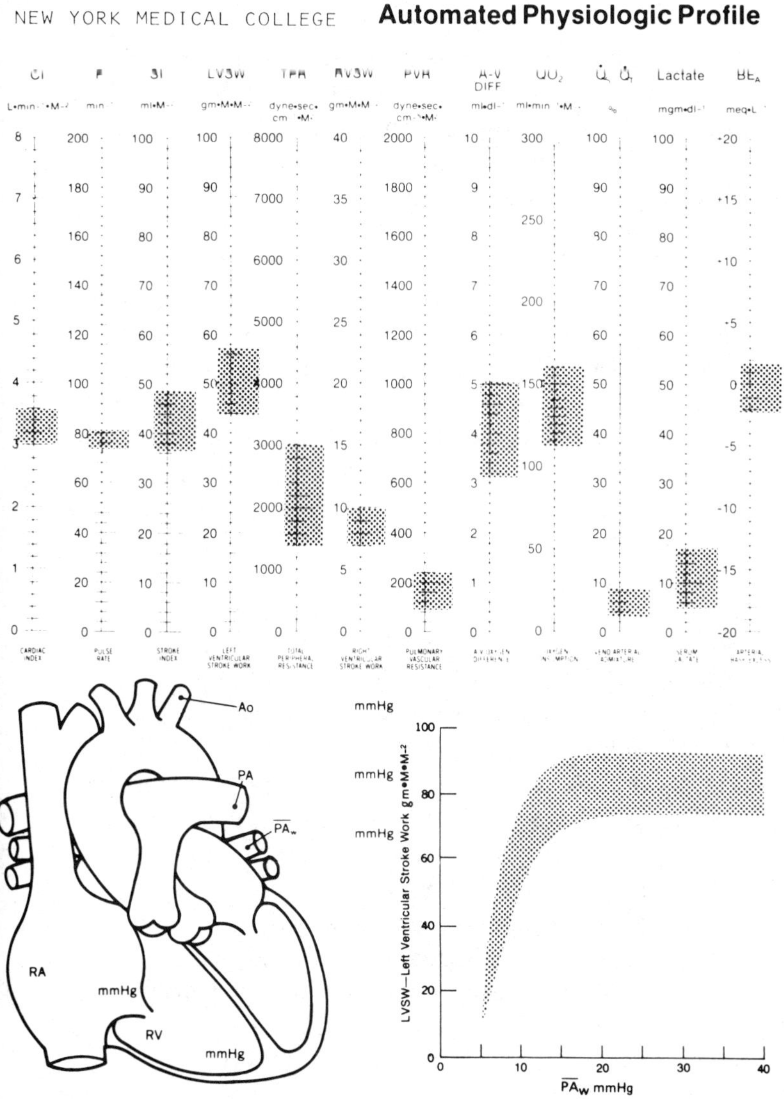

Figure 3-8. Automated physiologic profile, Reproduced, with permission, from Hospital Physician 13(10):12, October 1977

Serum lactate level. The serum lactate level indicates whether oxygen transport is sufficient for cellular metabolism. Normal metabolism requires oxygen; if oxygen supplies are decreased, anaerobic metabolism will dominate. A by-product of anaerobic metabolism is lactate, which will increase above the normal level of 2 mEq/L. The serum lactate level is a good gauge of the shock patient's probable survival.[5]

Monitoring derived parameters. There are various methods for obtaining and displaying the derived parameters commonly monitored for the patient in shock. Formulas (Appendix 3-2) can be used once direct parameters have been measured, but this can be time-consuming. Some critical care units utilize hand-held calculators that can quickly calculate derived variables. Another method is the automated physiologic profile, which displays derived variables on an easily scanned bar-chart format.[8]

The automated physiologic profile is a permanent record of the patient's cardiorespiratory and oxygen transport status. Patient data—such as PA and PAW pressures, height, weight, cardiac output, hemoglobin, and lactate—are entered into a computer. The computer then presents, on a preprinted format, the patient's primary and derived data, with the range of normal values for each parameter. A ventricular function curve is also constructed on the profile. The profile can easily be obtained and is used to assess both degree of shock and response to specific therapies such as vasopressors, positive inotropic agents, and PEEP.

Figure 3-8 is an automated physiologic profile of a patient in cardiogenic shock. Note the presence of diminished CI, SI, and LVSW and high PAW pressure, which reflect impaired LV function. The ventricular function curve also reveals poor ventricular performance. The pulse rate and SVR are increased as compensatory mechanisms. The patient's a-vDO_2 and serum lactate are high, verifying inadequate oxygen to meet the tissues' needs. This patient was successfully treated with intraaortic balloon counterpulsation.

Summary

Monitoring of the patient in shock presents a unique challenge to the critical care nurse, who must integrate complex data—obtained through physical assessment, directly measured parameters, and derived calculations—with the patient's underlying pathology in order to provide adequate care. No single measurement or group of parameters is sufficient. Accurate assessment of the shock patient's cardiorespiratory and oxygen transport status demands continuous monitoring of all the factors discussed in this chapter.

REFERENCES

1. Shoemaker W, Czer L: Evaluation of the biologic importance of various hemodynamic and oxygen transport variables: Which variables should be monitored in postoperative shock? *Crit Care Med* 7:424, 1979

2. Vij D, Babcock R, Magilligan D: A simplified concept of complete physiologic monitoring of the critically ill patient. *Heart Lung* 10:75, 1981

3. Daily E, Schroeder J: *Techniques in Bedside Hemodynamic Monitoring,* 2nd ed, p 35. St Louis: Mosby, 1981

4. Guyton A: *Textbook of Medical Physiology,* 5th ed, p 267. Philadelphia: Saunders, 1976

5. DelGurcio L, Kazarian K: Monitoring the patient in shock. *Hosp Phys* 77:12, 1977

6. Bodai B, Holcroft J: Use of the pulmonary arterial catheter in the critically ill patient. *Heart Lung* 11:406, 1982

7. Riedinger M, Shellock F, Swan H: Reading pulmonary artery and pulmonary capillary wedge pressure waveforms with respiratory variations. *Heart Lung* 10:675, 1981

8. Cohn J, Engler P, DelGurcio L: The automated physiologic profile. *Crit Care Med* 3:51, 1975

Appendix 3-1. Parameters Monitored in Shock: Abbreviations and Norms

PARAMETER	ABBREVIATION	NORMAL VALUE	UNITS
Arteriovenous oxygen difference	$a\text{-}vDO_2$	3.0-5.5	vol%
Cardiac index	CI	2.5-4.0	$L/min/m^2$
Cardiac output	CO	4.0-8.0	L/min
Central venous pressure	CVP	2-6	mm Hg
Left ventricular end-diastolic pressure	LVEDP	5-12	mm Hg
Left ventricular stroke work	LVSW	45-85	$g\text{-}m/m^2$
Mean arterial pressure	MAP	100	mm Hg
Pulmonary artery pressure	PAP	$\frac{20 = 30/10 = 20}{10 = 15}$	mm Hg
Pulmonary artery wedge pressure	PAWP	4-12	mm Hg
Right atrial pressure	RAP	2-6	mm Hg
Stroke index	SI	35-70	$mL/beat/m^2$
Stroke volume	SV	60-130	mL/beat
Systemic vascular resistance	SVR	900-1600	$dyne/sec/cm^5$

Appendix 3-2. Formulas for Calculating Derived Parameters

1. Arteriovenous oxygen difference:
   $a\text{-}vDO_2$ = arterial O_2 content − venous O_2 content

2. Cardiac index:

$$CI = \frac{CO}{BSA\ (m^2)}$$

3. Left ventricular stroke work:

$$LVSW = \frac{\frac{CI\ (MAP\ -\ PAWP)}{13.6}}{HR}$$

4. Mean arterial pressure:

$$MAP = \frac{\text{systolic blood pressure} - 2\ (\text{diastolic pressure})}{3}$$

5. Oxygen content:

$$O_2\ \text{content (vol\%)} = \%\ \text{sat} \times Hb \times 1.34$$

6. Stroke index:

$$SI = \frac{CI \times 1{,}000}{HR}$$

7. Systemic vascular resistance:

$$SVR = \frac{(MAP - RA)79.9}{CO}$$

4

HYPOVOLEMIC SHOCK

ANN M. PETLIN, RN, BSN, CCRN
and
JACQUELINE M. CAROLAN, RN, BSN, CCRN

The nature of shock is outlined at the beginning of Chapter 1. This chapter considers the syndrome of hypovolemic shock, probably the most common type, which is generally associated with other causes of decreased tissue perfusion.

Etiology

Hypovolemic shock is initiated by a loss of circulating fluid, which may result from decreased body water, hemorrhage or obstruction, or plasma shifts.

Decreased body water. In cardiogenic and septic shock, fluid loss is due to another primary pathology (heart disease or infection). Other causes of fluid loss include prolonged vomiting and diarrhea, heat exhaustion, diabetic acidosis, adrenal insufficiency, diabetes insipidus, and excessive use of diuretics. In infants and small children, the commonest cause of hypovolemic shock is diarrhea.

Hemorrhage or obstruction. Hemorrhage, whether from trauma or gastrointestinal bleeding, results in the loss of whole blood. Occasionally, pregnancy will cause obstruction of the inferior vena cava, leading to venous obstruction and a decrease in circulating whole blood.

Plasma shifts. Thermal burns cause shifts of plasma fluids as a result of increased capillary permeability in burned and unburned tissue. Most patients with burns on more than 25% of the total body surface will develop hypovolemia.

Pathophysiology

Compensatory mechanisms allow the body to lose up to 10% of circulating fluid while remaining relatively asymptomatic. When the circulating volume drops to between 15 and 25% of normal, symptoms of hypoperfusion begin to appear. In most cases, there is a drop in blood pressure that essentially reflects reduced cardiac output and peripheral resistance. The blood pressure consists of three parts: (1) diastolic pressure, which correlates with the amount of vasoconstriction; (2) pulse pressure (the difference between systolic and diastolic pressures), which reflects the rigidity of the aorta and relates to stroke volume; and (3) systolic pressure, which is determined by a combination of these factors. In hypovolemic shock, decreases in stroke volume and pulse pressure usually occur before there is a significant fall in systolic pressure. With hemorrhage, sympathoadrenal stimulation causes vasoconstriction, and diastolic pressure generally rises initially. The total peripheral resistance also rises to compensate for the reduction in cardiac output. The organs that are most affected by the increase in peripheral resistance are the skin and the kidneys.

Along with the changes already mentioned, an increase in pulse rate will be seen with a reduction in circulating blood volume. This is due to a compensatory sympathetic response. Since so many variables affect pulse rate, the degree of increase is not an absolute value; but observation of pulse rate becomes significant in evaluating response to therapy.

Endogenous hemodilution

In the initial phases of hypovolemia or hypotension, fluids tend to move from the interstitial space into the vascular compartment as a normal homeostatic response. In patients with hypovolemia due to hemorrhage, this response is reflected in the hematocrit. In the early, acute stage of hemorrhage, the hematocrit will be normal because the patient has lost proportional amounts of red cells and plasma. After transcapillary refill of the vascular space, the hematocrit drops. Intravascular volume may be reestablished and the blood pressure near normal, but there are still inadequate red blood cells available to carry oxygen and nutrients.

Metabolic and respiratory alterations

Patients with trauma or shock tend to hyperventilate early, causing respiratory alkalosis. These patients tend to have minute volumes $1\frac{1}{2}$ to 2 times normal. Before shock, respiratory alkalosis is a nonspecific response; later in shock, respiratory alkalosis is a compensation for metabolic acidosis. Metabolic acidosis is due mainly to the accumulation of lactic acid in late and severe hemorrhagic shock. Ordinarily, pyruvic acid, a normal product of glycolysis, enters the Krebs cycle, leading to the production of high-energy phosphate bonds. In hemorrhagic shock, oxygen delivery to the cells declines. Since the entry of pyruvate into the Krebs cycle is oxygen-dependent, pyruvate levels in the plasma rise during shock. Part of the excess pyruvate is converted to lactic acid, a strong organic acid. It has been shown that, in the shock state, lactic acid elevation occurs before a clinical drop in blood pressure is apparent. A decrease in lacticemia reflects a favorable response to therapy.

As already stated, most patients in hemorrhagic shock have an abnormal pattern of breathing; they must work harder to achieve alveolar ventilation, either because of greater airway resistance or increased lung stiffness. This stiffness may be related to increased interstitial sodium and water in the lungs.

Skin changes

The patient in shock may first experience piloerection (gooseflesh) as blood is shunted away from the extremities. However, the intense sympathoadrenal stimulation of hypovolemic shock can prompt a progression to generalized cold, clammy skin. If this is observed, the patient probably has both a low cardiac output and a high systemic vascular resistance. This is usually a late sign. In certain forms of septic or cardiogenic shock, the skin may be relatively warm and dry. Flushing and sweating at any time indicate overheating, which increases the metabolic rate and need for oxygen.

Sensorium

The body's compensatory mechanisms during shock are directed largely toward maintaining perfusion to the brain, heart, and kidneys. These patients may complain of a feeling of impending doom before any clinical change can be detected. Confusion, drowsiness, disorientation, and increasing lethargy are all signs of poor perfusion to the brain. There may also be muscle weakness, as metabolism is forced into anaerobic pathways and lactic acid levels rise.

Temperature

With hemorrhagic shock, the body temperature often drops below normal. Therefore, such patients should be covered with a light blanket so that energy is conserved as they try to keep warm. A gradually increasing temperature may indicate atelectasis due to hypoventilation or developing sepsis. A person with hypovolemia due to heat exhaustion may be febrile because not enough body water for normal cooling mechanisms is available.

Urine output

There is usually a good correlation between urine output and renal blood flow, which is dependent on cardiac output. When cardiac output is reduced by severe hypovolemia, urinary output usually falls as well. If the fall in renal blood flow is more gradual, urinary sodium falls and urinary osmolality rises before urine output drops. Here the kidneys are attempting to conserve water by reabsorbing more sodium and excreting a more concentrated urine.

Because shock is a clinically dynamic state, it is important that the patient receive thorough and continuous assessment. No one laboratory value or physical measurement is sufficient to indicate the patient's degree of illness. Instead, sets of data must be evaluated for the development of trends and correlated with the patient's actual clinical state.

Blood pressure monitoring

Arterial pressure

Arterial blood pressure is a good guide to therapy, and is covered in Chapter 3.

The noninvasive Doppler technique is an acceptable alternative to continuous intraarterial pressure measurements because it provides accurate estimates of systolic pressure long after Korotkoff's sounds are inaudible.

Venous pressure

Measurements of central venous pressure (CVP) are important because fluid loss leads to decreased pressure in the venous vascular bed. This eventually decreases the filling pressure of the right ventricle and is reflected in the CVP. The CVP is extremely variable in critically ill patients; it may not accurately reflect the patient's fluid losses and volume requirements. However, monitoring of the pulmonary artery (with a floating balloon catheter) is of significant help in the management of shock, as discussed in Chapter 3. The pulmonary artery wedge pressure (PAWP), or pulmonary capillary wedge pressure, reflects the function of the left heart more accurately and is more sensitive to fluid overload than the CVP. The CVP and/or PAWP are important in evaluating the effects of fluid replacement in the patient with hypovolemic shock.

Measurement of cardiac output

Cardiac output is measured most conveniently by use of the balloon-tipped, flow-directed thermodilution (Swan-Ganz) catheter. It can also be measured through the administration of an indicator dye that is sensed by special light-sensitive monitors. Cardiac output is a more sensitive measurement of adequate tissue perfusion than is blood pressure. When the circulating blood volume falls, the cardiac output usually drops as well. In early phases of hypovolemic shock, cardiac output may be normal or even above normal because of sympathoadrenal stimulation.

A urine output below 30mL/h is usually a sign of decreased perfusion of the kidneys and the rest of the body's tissues. Specific gravity can easily be checked at the patient's bedside. If it is greater than 1.020, the patient is probably fluid-depleted and the kidneys are functioning normally in their efforts to conserve fluids. The urine osmolality is a more accurate reflection of renal concentrating ability. For patients who remain critically ill, daily weights are a more sensitive indication of fluid loss or gain than are intake/output measurements. Intake/output records should be compared with daily weight determinations in order to check for insensible fluid losses, fluid shifts, or errors in calculations.

Laboratory studies

As already mentioned, the hematocrit is normal in the early stages of hypovolemia due to hemorrhagic trauma. When transcapillary refill occurs, the hematocrit drops. When the hematocrit is below 30%, there is a significant reduction of oxygen-carrying capacity to cells that are already suffering from poor perfusion. The hematocrit guides the physician in choosing blood products (whole blood or packed cells) and colloids versus electrolyte solutions. An elevated white blood cell count is a normal response to stress. As illness continues, however, an elevated white blood cell count should arouse suspicion of developing infection.

Blood gases. Blood gases provide essential information about respiratory function and acid-base balance. The arterial PO_2 (normal, 80 to 100 mm Hg) indicates the level of oxygenation. Early phases of shock are characterized by respiratory alkalosis, with a decreased arterial PCO_2 (normal, 35 to 45 mm Hg). Combined with low pH (normal, 7.39 to 7.41) and bicarbonate levels (normal, 20 to 24 mEq/L), this indicates that the patient is attempting to make respiratory compensation for the developing metabolic acidosis.

Electrolytes. Serum electrolytes provide information about abnormalities caused by shock. An elevated serum sodium (normal, 135 to 145 mEq/L) may indicate hypovolemia due to dehydration. As complications set in, or as a result of treatment, other abnormalities may occur. An elevated serum potassium (normal, 3.5 to 5.0 mEq/L) may follow the administration of large amounts of blood. Potassium may also rise in acute renal failure.

Serum osmolality. Serum osmolality (normal, 285 to 290) provides information on the patient's state of hydration and may guide the choice of fluids for volume replacement. When compared with urine osmolality, it also assesses renal function. Blood urea nitrogen (normal, 7 to 25 mg/100 mL) and creatinine (normal, 0.5 to 1.5 mg/100 mL) also contribute data on the kidneys.

Serum lactate and pyruvate. Serum lactate or serum pyruvate levels are monitored at some hospitals. Normal serum lactate is 5 to 15 mg/100 mL. Both lactate and pyruvate levels rise as anaerobic metabolism increases, and these levels correlate fairly well with the degree of shock. When arterial lactate levels approach 80 mg/100 mL, there is a marked decrease in survival.

Electrocardiogram. ECG monitoring, done continuously at bedside, should be provided for the patient in shock when possible. Thus tachycardias or other arrhythmias can be detected early. The 12-lead ECG may show nonspecific ST segment or T wave changes in the hypovolemic patient as a result of decreased coronary blood flow. Chest x-rays may be ordered to assess the patient's pulmonary status.

Treatment

The primary goal of treatment of hypovolemic shock is to anticipate it and prevent its occurrence. The earlier that the suspicion of developing shock is raised, the more likely it is that the patient will receive appropriate assessment and treatment. In fact, many emergency departments consider trauma patients to be in hypovolemic shock until proven otherwise.

Maintaining vital signs. Many patients escape early evaluation or do not appear until shock is in progress. The goals of treatment then are initially the same as those for every critically ill patient: to maintain an open airway, assure that the patient is breathing, and maintain cardiac and cerebral circulation. Once these are met, the next goal is to restore an effective circulating volume.

Replacing fluids. Electrolyte solutions are usually the first choice for volume replacement. The primary electrolyte replacement solutions are physiologic saline (0.9% sodium chloride solution) and Ringer's lactate. Ringer's lactate is usually the preferred solution because its electrolyte content closely resembles that of extracellular fluid. With normal liver function, the lactate is converted to bicarbonate ion. This may help to correct the underlying acidosis.

The amount of fluid replaced is critical, since fluid overload may cause congestive heart failure. Excessive amounts of electrolyte solution given without colloids may cause pulmonary edema by decreasing the colloid osmotic pressure. For an adult patient with clinical signs of hypovolemia, 2 to 3 L of normal saline or Ringer's lactate are infused over an hour. Blood pressure, pulse, urine output, skin color, and sensorium are checked frequently. If they don't improve, the patient may be losing circulating volume faster than it can be replaced; surgery may have to be considered.

If the patient remains hypovolemic after administration of crystalloid solutions, colloids may be given.

Replacing blood, platelets, or plasma. In cases of hemorrhagic shock, it is obvious that blood is needed. However, whole blood is transfused only for massive hemorrhage in an emergency, when components are unavailable. To improve the hemoglobin and hematocrit, packed red blood cells are preferred because they carry less risk of overload, are less likely to transmit hepatitis, and contain less sodium, potassium, ammonium, and citrate. One unit of packed cells raises the hematocrit approximately 3 percentage points.

Fresh frozen plasma can be given as a volume expander, especially to patients with liver insufficiency when there are several coexisting deficiency factors. To restore or maintain blood volume in hypovolemia without acute blood loss, the plasma volume expander of choice is albumin. It does not carry hepatitis, and 50 mL of 25% albumin have the osmotic effect of 1 unit of plasma. Dextran, a hypertonic colloidal solution, is also an excellent plasma expander. It produces an immediate, though brief, expansion of plasma volume by drawing fluid from interstitial to intravascular spaces. Dextran is also beneficial in that it retards and reverses cellular aggregation resulting from shock.

Since all of these products have pharmacologic as well as mechanical properties, they must be given carefully and side effects watched for.

Drug therapy

When patients remain in shock after apparently adequate fluid resuscitation, drugs must be considered.

Dopamine. Dopamine (Intropin) is currently the initial drug of choice. In low doses (2 to 5 μg/kg/min), it increases urine output by diluting the renal vascular bed. In moderate doses (5 to 20 μg/kg/min); it increases cardiac output by inotropic stimulation. High doses (above 20 μg/kg/min) should be avoided. At these levels, severe peripheral vasoconstriction results and cellular blood flow is impaired even more.

Isoproterenol. Isoproterenol (Isuprel) increases cardiac output and reduces peripheral vascular resistance when given in doses below 2 μg/min. Its usefulness is limited by the tachycardia it produces, which decreases diastolic filling time.

Digitalis. Digitalis preparations may be used to improve cardiac performance. Serum potassium and calcium levels must be monitored during digitalis therapy to avoid cardiac arrhythmias.

Dobutamine. Dobutamine (Dobutrex) is used in the short-term treatment of adults with cardiac decompensation due to depressed contractility. It increases cardiac output without a marked increase in heart rate.

Norepinephrine. Norepinephrine (Levophed) is a sympathomimetic drug that produces powerful vasoconstriction and stimulation of the heart and dilation of the coronary arteries. However, vasopressors can cause almost complete occlusion of arterioles, causing a decrease of blood flow to larger tissue areas. Therefore, if blood pressure is adequate, a vasodilator such as nitroglycerin or sodium nitroprusside (Nipride) could probably be given as well, in order to modify the vasoconstrictive effect.

Corticosteroids. Corticosteroids are used more commonly in septic shock than in hypovolemic shock. They help to protect cell membranes and decrease the inflammatory response to stress. Peripheral blood flow to poorly perfused organs may be promoted by steroidal effects on peripheral vasodilation. The sodium and water retention caused by corticosteroids may help to correct the hypovolemia.

Epinephrine. Epinephrine (Adrenalin) may be used for its cardiostimulatory and peripheral vasoconstrictive effects. Peripheral vasoconstriction is usually maximal in shock, however, and further constriction may be detrimental. For the same reason, metaraminol (Aramine) is rarely used in hypovolemic shock.

Additional treatments

Oxygen. Adequate oxygenation is essential to a patient in shock. Oxygen via a mask or nasal cannula may be an adequate supplement. The level of oxygenation is reflected in the arterial blood gases (ABGs). If the ABGs indicate a greater need for ventilatory support, the patient may require intubation and artificial ventilation on a respirator. By manipulating ventilator settings for oxygen, tidal volume, and respiratory rate, both oxygen and acid-base imbalances may be treated.

Bicarbonate. Metabolic acidosis is often corrected as soon as cellular perfusion is improved. If acidosis persists in spite of adequate fluid replacement, the patient may require sodium bicarbonate. When bicarbonate is given cautiously, it improves the action of other drugs by optimizing the acid-base level. Organ performance is also enhanced.

Bicarbonate must be given with care, since excessive amounts can cause metabolic alkalosis. The sodium bicarbonate solution is hypertonic and may affect serum osmolarity. The high sodium load may also cause excess fluid retention and contribute to heart failure.

Mannitol. If the patient is receiving adequate fluids, specific treatment for renal support may not be necessary. If urine output drops below 30 to 50 mL/h, 12.5 to

25 g of mannitol may be given intravenously. This osmotic diuretic pulls fluid into the intravascular space. Both mannitol and water are then extracted and excreted as they pass through the kidneys. Mannitol may protect cell membranes as well.

Furosemide. If mannitol does not adequately increase urine output, 5 to 10 mg of furosemide (Lasix) may be given intravenously. This powerful loop diuretic acts by inhibiting the action of certain renal cells, enhancing both potassium and fluid excretion. However, no diuretic can prevent renal failure if the underlying cause of the problem is not treated.

Nutritional support. The shock state places increased demands on the body. Anaerobic metabolism is less energy-efficient than aerobic metabolism. Calories stored within the body in the form of glucose and glycogen are exhausted early. Hypovolemia may decrease blood flow to the digestive system and lower the absorption of nutrients. Because of these factors, nutritional assessment and support should begin promptly. Some medical centers begin to administer high-calorie glucose solutions (50% dextrose) early in the course of therapy for shock. Parenteral or enteral nutrition may provide beneficial support for patients in this severe state of stress.

Nursing measures

Nursing measures are a valuable adjunct to the medical management of shock. Attention to psychological needs is important. Because these patients are under great stress, such attention may actually affect their response to treatment.

Psychological support. The patient in shock is usually frightened and often helpless; therefore, procedures should be explained simply before they are carried out. And because nonverbal communication is as important as verbal, a gentle touch and reassuring attitude may also help calm the patient. Family and friends should be allowed regular visits to provide reassurance in an otherwise overwhelming environment.

Recognizing that family members may also be under stress, offer them support as well. Periodic explanations of the patient's condition and treatment may help allay some fears.

Physical support. When the patient is positioned flat in bed, both cardiac and cerebral circulation are promoted. The patient may still be turned from side to side, but avoid the Trendelenburg position, as it increases respiratory impairment.

Because the patient is using a great deal of energy just to meet physiologic needs, measures to conserve energy are implemented. A quiet environment is ideal but nearly impossible when the patient is so critically ill. Plan nursing care to allow for periods of rest, however brief. The patient should be moved to other departments or diagnostic areas only when absolutely necessary.

Aseptic technique. Because shock patients are under stress, their immune response is impaired. Therefore, the entire health care team must pay especially strict attention to aseptic technique.

Record keeping. Finally, it is important to maintain precise records. As mentioned earlier, no one observation or measurement provides significant information about the patient. Rather, it is the trends reflected by these data and their correlation with the patient's clinical condition that indicate how successful the therapies have been.

The use of external counterpressure

Hemorrhage, both internal and external, is the most common cause of hypovolemic shock seen in the emergency department. External pressure over bleeding sites is often the only way to control bleeding until the patient can be prepared for surgery.

Control of bleeding

The rate of blood loss after trauma depends both on the size of the break in the artery or vein and on the pressure within the vessel. When pressure between the inside and outside of the vessel is decreased by external counterpressure, the elastic tissue in the arterial wall retracts and the diameter of the artery decreases. This slows bleeding and may bring about hemostasis. External pressure as low as 20 to 25 mm Hg will help even in arterial bleeds.

The pressure needed to empty the venous system is low; 5 to 15 mm Hg of counterpressure bring about nearly complete emptying. Some believe that no more than 25 mm Hg of counterpressure is needed for any reason. Even this low pressure has been shown to be effective in treatment of massive bleeds.

The antishock suit

In 1903, it was proposed that application of circumferential counterpressure to the lower extremities with a device that surrounds the legs and pelvis would prevent pooling of venous blood and promote hemostasis of bleeding sites. Eventually, a special pressurized suit was developed—a modification of one worn by aviators that prevents pooling of blood in the lower extremities during high-acceleration maneuvers. Currently, two models are available: the military antishock trousers, or MAST suit, and the Gladiator antishock airpants. These vary in the placement of the Velcro closures and in the use of a monitoring valve that indicates pressure within the suit.

Function. External pressure on the venous system of the legs and pelvis increases the return of blood to the heart. When the antishock suit is applied, the venous system in the lower body is almost completely emptied. In essence, the patient receives an autotransfusion of blood from his own venous pools. An improvement in the patient's condition after application of the suit supports a diagnosis of hypovolemia.

Uses. Besides being useful in bleeding and hypovolemia, the antishock suit can be used to help splint lower extremity and pelvic fractures. Ruptured ectopic pregnancy and major abdominal bleeds may be treated initially by applying the suit. The onset of hypovolemic shock can be delayed if the suit is applied early.

Application. To apply the antishock suit, the patient is first placed upon it. Areas of the legs and pelvis going into the suit are examined closely, and the Velcro closures then are wrapped around the legs and pelvis. Separate valves control inflation of the bladders surrounding each section. The leg bladders are inflated first. This helps to push blood from the lower extremities up toward the central organs. The section covering the pelvis is inflated last, in order to promote emptying of the pelvic veins.

Monitoring. Assess the patient's blood pressure, pulse, and sensorium frequently. The improvement in blood pressure, decrease in tachycardia, and clearing of the sensorium after application of the suit are often dramatic. In cases of bleeding from the pelvis or lower extremities, this approach may provide stability until surgery can begin. On the other hand, localized hemostasis may suffice to make surgery unnecessary.

Once the antishock suit is on, it should remain in place until the patient can receive adequate treatment. That is, the patient should be transported to x-ray or surgery in the garment, and x-rays can be taken through it. The suit also provides access to the perineum for insertion of urinary catheters. The limb leads for a 12-lead ECG can be placed by releasing small areas of the leg sections.

Frequently check peripheral pulses in the patient's feet to assure that the external pressure has not occluded arterial flow.

Removal. After receiving treatment, the patient must be weaned from the trousers by releasing pressure from the bladders gradually. A drop in blood pressure of 5 mm Hg or more indicates too rapid deflation. Large-gauge intravenous lines should already be in place in case rapid volume replacement should be required after release of external counterpressure. The pelvic section of the trousers is deflated first, to prevent a tourniquet effect on the legs.

Possible side effects. Side effects of the trousers are related to the amount of pressure applied. Respiratory acidosis may develop if the antishock suit restricts ventilation. Lacticacidosis may develop because there is decreased perfusion to cells of the lower extremities while the suit is in place.

Contraindications. The only absolute contraindications for the use of this treatment are congestive heart failure and pulmonary edema, where the patient's heart has difficulty handling increased volumes of blood. Other possible contraindications are pneumothorax or hemothorax and increased intracranial pressure. Such cases must await the physician's judgment. In pregnancy, application of the pelvic section may be hazardous, but trauma and the risk of shock may be even more dangerous to the mother and fetus. Obstetric departments have made successful use of the antishock suit with women who were suffering from massive postpartum hemorrhage.

BIBLIOGRAPHY

Bryan-Brown C, et al: In *Principles and Techniques of Critical Care.* Kalamazoo, Mich: The Upjohn Company, 1979

Pelligra R: Outside pressure for an inside bleed. *Emerg Med* 11(8):24, August 1979

Pepine CJ, et al: Guidelines for evaluation and management of shock. *Hosp Med* 15(3):88, March 1979

Zamora BO: Management of hemorrhagic shock. *Hosp Med* 15(7):6, July 1979

5

SEPTIC SHOCK

GLORIA OBLOUK DAROVIC, RN, CCRN

Septic shock may develop from any infectious disease, whether caused by viruses, spirochetes, parasites, rickettsiae, fungi, gram-positive bacteria, or gram-negative bacteria. Although gram-negative bacteria are by far the most common causative agents, staphylococci, streptococci, pneumococci, and clostridia can also produce shock states. (The term septic shock usually used synonymously with endotoxic shock, gram-negative sepsis, bacterial shock, bacteremic shock, septicemic shock, endotoxemia, and septicemia.)[1]

During the past 25 to 30 years, the incidence of septic shock has increased approximately 20 times, making it a major threat to hospitalized patients.[2] This chapter covers its epidemiology and pathogenesis, pathophysiology, treatment, and prevention.

Epidemiology and pathogenesis

Development of antibiotic-resistant organisms

Since their introduction in the 1940s, antibiotics have had the paradoxical effect of promoting some types of bacterial infections. In greatly reducing the number of gram-positive organisms in an infected patient (the major source of infections), these "miracle drugs" cleared the way for opportunistic, ever-present, gram-negative bacteria. The latter showed a unique ability to develop antibiotic-resistant strains and were thus able to multiply where their former competitors no longer could. This tendency was further encouraged by the indiscriminate and incorrect use of antibiotics, until eventually bacterial resistance to antibiotic drugs became a major medical dilemma. Wherever antibiotics are commonly used, as in the modern hospital, resistant gram-negative bacteria prevail. Further, most of the infected patients are in the critical care areas.[3, 4]

Table 5-1. Factors Favoring Septic Shock

INADEQUATE IMMUNE RESPONSE	PRIMARY INFECTIONS
Granulocytopenia	Pneumonia
Diabetes mellitus	Genitourinary infections
Liver disease	Cholecystitis
Neoplasms	Peritonitis
Early infancy	Iatrogenic sources
Extreme old age	Indwelling vascular catheters
Alcoholism	Indwelling urinary catheters
Renal failure	Instrumentation of the urinary tract
Pregnancy	Extensive surgery, especially abdominal or pelvic
Malnutrition	

Invasive procedures

The incidence of gram-negative sepsis in hospitals is also favored by the development of complex, invasive, diagnostic and surgical procedures, especially in elderly or debilitated patients who are ready hosts for infection. Indwelling tubes or catheters offer easy access to bacterial invaders. Instrumentation such as cystoscopy carries the same risk. Likewise, structural damage or distortion of organs eases the penetration of mucosal barriers by infectious organisms.[1]

Immunosuppression and old age

The most favorable host for gram-negative sepsis is elderly and has an impaired immune system. Except for those who are pregnant or immunosuppressed, patients below age 40 rarely develop hypotension and "cold shock."[5]

Trauma

Finally, trauma is an important predisposing factor. For example, the presence of blood in the peritoneal cavity greatly increases the likelihood of peritonitis, because hemoglobin impairs the phagocytic activity of the white blood cells and also competes with them for oxygen. And trauma patients, particularly if they have been in shock, are at greater risk for infection because of impairment of their immune systems.

Table 5-1 summarizes these and other factors favoring the development of septic shock.

Mortality

In spite of voluminous research into the management of septic shock, the mortality ranges from 40 to 80% in most institutions.[3, 4] These high rates are explained at least partly by the fact that the typical septic shock patient already has serious underlying disease that may have compromised the function of the vital organs.

Gram-positive and gram-negative organisms

Various gram-positive organisms normally live on the skin and the mucous membranes. When some of these infect a host, they liberate a protein toxin as a by-product of their metabolism. This passes through the organism's cell wall and is therefore called an exotoxin; it causes the signs and symptoms of the specific disease. For example, it is the powerful exotoxin of *Clostridium botulinum* that causes paralysis and death in botulism food poisoning (see Table 5-2).

Many of the gram-negative bacteria inhabiting our bodies live on the skin and in the upper respiratory tract; however, they reside mainly in the intestines. Most of

Table 5-2. Some Diseases Caused by Gram-Positive Organisms

ORGANISM	DISEASE
Staphylococcus aureus	Wound infection Impetigo
Beta-hemolytic streptococci	Tonsillitis Rheumatic fever Neonatal infections Puerperal infections
Klebsiella pneumoniae (Diplococcus pneumoniae)	Pneumonia Paranasal infections Middle ear infections Meningitis
Clostridium tetani	Tetanus
Clostridium perfringens	Gas gangrene
Clostridium botulinum	Botulism
Corynebacterium diphtheriae	Diphtheria

them are harmless and actually contribute to health by competing with disease-causing organisms that may produce diarrhea and other gastrointestinal disturbances. They also play a role in the utilization of certain vitamins. Common among the normal intestinal flora are *Escherichia coli, Clostridium perfringens, Bacteroides, Lactobacillus acidophilus,* and members of the *Pseudomonas* and *Proteus* groups. Their presence outside their normal environment can cause infections, such as peritonitis and cystitis.

The gram-negative organism harbors its toxin within the cell wall—hence the term endotoxin—and releases it only upon death. When the gram-negative organisms remain within their normal environment, their endotoxins cause no harm. However, when they contaminate other body structures or cavities, endotoxin release becomes potentially lethal.

Outside the body, any source of moisture favors the growth and residence of gram-negative bacteria. Humidifiers, sinks, mechanical ventilators, irrigation fluids, and potted or cut flowers are all possible sources of contamination (see Table 5-3).

Pathophysiology

When circulating gram-negative bacilli release their endotoxins into the blood as a result of disruption of their cell walls by the antimicrobial effects of antibiotics or phagocytosis, "these macromolecules are read by our tissues as the very worst of bad news."[6] Ironically, it is not so much the direct effect of the toxin on the body but the body's explosive and exaggerated defense reaction to it that produces widespread tissue destruction and death.

This mechanism, which distinguishes septic shock from shock due to other causes, has come to be understood only within the past 20 years. Previously, it was felt that the signs and symptoms of all forms of shock were due to underperfusion at the microcirculatory level,

Table 5-3. Some Diseases Caused by Gram-Negative Organisms

ORGANISM	DISEASE
Neisseria gonorrhoeae	Gonorrhea
Neisseria meningitidis	Epidemic meningitis
Salmonella typhi	Typhoid fever
Haemophilus influenzae	Upper respiratory infection
	Middle ear infection
	Epiglottitis
	Meningitis (in children under 3)

	Cardiac output	Peripheral vascular resistance
Early	↑	↓
Late	↓	↑

Figure 5-1 Cardiovascular responses in gram-negative septic shock

which, in turn, stemmed from low cardiac output, hypotension, and increased resistance to the flow of blood due to vasoconstriction.

More recently, however, it has been found that septic shock has two distinct, time-related phases. In the early phase, the patient's cardiovascular system is in a hyperdynamic state; as septicemia progresses, a hypodynamic state supervenes.[7, 8] The hyperdynamic phase may last from minutes to hours, depending on the quantity and virulence of the infecting agents as well as on host resistance. With early and effective therapy, the hypodynamic phase, or "cold shock," may never appear.

Hyperdynamic phase

Blood flow. During this phase, marked by vasodilation and decreased peripheral vascular resistance (Figure 5-1), the blood pressure is normal or only slightly decreased. Cardiac output is increased, as a compensatory mechanism, to maintain blood pressure despite the enlarged vascular bed. Because the capillaries become permeable, the liquid portion of the blood tends to leak into the interstitial spaces (third-space losses)—a phenomenon that can result in the loss of more than 200 mL/h of circulating fluid. At this point, therefore, the patient begins to develop hypovolemia because of the increased size of the vascular bed and third-space losses. The peripheral vasodilation and increased capillary permeability are thought to result from activation of the

Table 5-4. Signs and Symptoms of Septic Shock

EARLY: HYPERDYNAMIC PHASE	LATE: HYPODYNAMIC PHASE
Normotension or slight hypotension	Hypotension—may occur gradually or suddenly
Tachycardia; pulse may be bounding	Tachycardia; pulse weak and thready
Altered cerebral function manifested by restlessness, lethargy, changes in affect	Decreased level of consciousness
Skin warm, pink, and dry from vasodilation	Skin moist, cold, and pale with mottling and cyanosis
Hyperventilation—in the absence of pulmonary problems, should suggest sepsis in susceptible patients	Continued hyperventilation; with accumulation of lactic acid, metabolic acidosis prevails
Decreased central venous pressure, pulmonary artery pressure, and pulmonary artery wedge pressure; may be normal or elevated in left-sided heart failure	Pressures remain low, but may increase in left-sided heart failure Collapse of peripheral veins Oliguria and anuria
Decreased white cell count at first; then leukocytosis Fever; rarely hypothermia	Decreased bowel sounds; paralytic ileus may follow

complement- and bradykinin-generating systems triggered by endotoxin (see Table 5-4).

Skin color and temperature. The skin is warm, pink, and dry, owing to vasodilation. Fever is usually present, accompanied by shaking chills. In some cases, especially in the elderly or debilitated, temperature may drop below normal levels.

Breathing. Hyperventilation inappropriate to the body's need produces a respiratory alkalosis. This hyperventilation is thought to be due to stimulation of the respiratory centers directly by the endotoxin[9] and/or plugging of the pulmonary microvasculature by sticky, clumped white blood cells.[10]

Oxygenation. Despite the hyperventilation, there are signs of tissue hypoxia. These may appear as changes in cerebral function such as confusion, agitation, inappropriate behavior, or a dulled consciousness. The tissue hypoxia is thought to be due to the hemoglobin molecule's reluctance to give up oxygen to the cells as well as to the reduced ability of the endotoxin-compromised cells to take up and utilize the oxygen and nutrients brought to them. The derangements in oxygen delivery and uptake are thought to be due to endotoxin. Another school of thought holds that tissue hypoxia is due to arteriovenous shunting of blood past the capillary bed.

Other parameters. The white blood cell count, possibly low at first, bounds back quickly to leukocytosis. Urine output may fall. Central venous and pulmonary artery wedge pressures are normal to low.

Hypodynamic phase

Blood flow. When the cardiac output can no longer keep pace with the increasing expansion of the vascular space and fluid loss through leakage, hypotension develops. Peripheral vascular resistance is increased through the release of catecholamines, touched off by sympathetic nervous system stimulation in response to hypotension. Cardiac output progressively decreases for several possible reasons, including release of myocardial depressant factor, impaired myocardial metabolism, and myocardial ischemia due to impaired coronary perfusion. The pulse is weak and thready; ST and T wave changes may reflect inadequate coronary blood flow. The skin is cold, moist, and pale, with peripheral mottling and cyanosis. Oliguria may progress to anuria (Table 5-4). With the exception of fever, the patient presents the classic picture of shock.

Disseminated intravascular coagulation. Probably all patients in septic shock have hematologic abnormalities, frequently with clinical or laboratory evidence of disseminated intravascular coagulation (DIC). This condition begins when the endotoxin interacts with and initiates the coagulation mechanism. Coagulation is also initiated by the slow rate of blood flow. In addition, the bacteria—and/or the immune response to bacterial toxins—produce damage to the vascular endothelium, causing the adhesion of platelets and activation of the intrinsic coagulation system. These phenomena result in the formation of microthrombi and subsequent destruction of the microcirculation. DIC may also produce paradoxical hemorrhage through consumption of the coagulation factors (used in the manufacture of the multitudinous small clots) and secondary activation of the fibrinolytic system.

Oxygenation. Hypoxia due to impaired uptake and utilization of oxygen is now compounded by decreased perfusion at the microcirculatory level, perpetuating and augmenting shock. More tissues resort to metabolism via the anaerobic pathway, which results in the accumulation of lactic acid in the blood. This is reflected in blood gas studies as metabolic acidosis. In some laboratories, the arterial lactate can be measured (normal, 0.6 to 1.8 mEq/L). In hypoxia and shock, lacticacidemia is a measure of anaerobic tissue metabolism due to inadequate tissue oxygenation. If arterial lactate levels are not available, the base deficit done with standard blood gas analysis is a good indicator of oxidative metabolism. Normal base excess values are $+3$ to -3; a base excess below -5 mEq HCO_3/L indicates the presence of poor perfusion.[11]

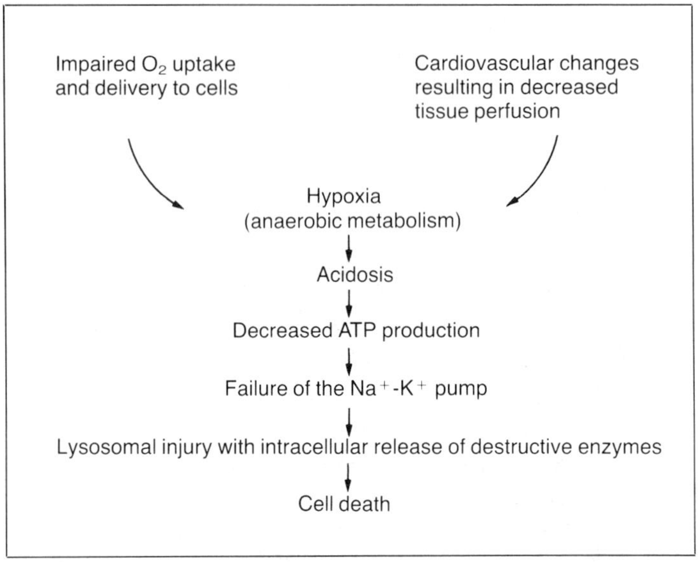

Figure 5-2 Sequence of events in irreversible septic shock (organ failure)

In addition to the accumulation of lactic acid, anaerobic metabolism is characterized by a 20-fold decrease in energy production. The acid environment, in combination with decreased energy production, further compromises cell function. There is a failure of the sodium-potassium pump mechanism and lysosomal breakdown, causing more cell dysfunction and death.

Organ failure. Ultimately, a stage is reached where tissue damage has become so devastating that the patient can no longer respond to therapy. This sequence of events is summarized in Figure 5-2.

Prevention

Septicemia always arises as a complication, never as a primary, spontaneously occurring disease. The predisposing factors are easily identified: a compromised host who has experienced an invasive procedure or organ damage. Preventive measures include the following and are the best "therapy" for septic shock:

1. Since it is impossible for gram-negative bacteria to grow in an absolutely dry environment, never let water stagnate in patients' rooms. This means the elimination of cut flowers, irrigation solutions, and so on. Dressings that are intended to be dry should be inspected frequently and kept dry.

2. Since indwelling urinary catheters can offer access to bacteria, handle them with care:

   a. Don't allow drainage bags to touch the floor.
   b. Don't disconnect the catheter from the drainage system, since breaks in the system may allow bacteria to enter.
   c. Don't raise the bag above the patient's bladder level, since this allows retrograde flow back to the bladder.
   d. Avoid irrigating a Foley catheter unless it's absolutely necessary. Use the irrigation equipment only once, then discard or resterilize it.
   e. Maintain good flow by guarding against obstructions in the tubing (kinks or compression).
   f. Give the catheterized patient a daily perineal wash with soap and water.

3. Intravenous catheters should not be allowed to remain in place longer than 72 hours, as the risk of infection increases with time. Dressings over puncture sites or wounds must be changed daily, using sterile technique and antimicrobial ointment.

4. Strict handwashing between patients, or when going from a dirty to a clean area in the same patient, is mandatory. This means a minimum of 30 seconds with the application of generous amounts of soap, water, and friction.

5. Sterile technique is essential in suctioning endotracheal tubes or tracheostomies.

6. Good oral hygiene should be maintained in the care of NPO or intubated patients. Without the periodic cleansing benefits of eating and drinking, bacteria multiply and accumulate in the oral cavity and pharynx. Apart from the risk of aspirating infected material, the mere proximity of a dirty oropharynx to the sterile lungs carries a high risk of pulmonary contamination.

Treatment

The treatment of established sepsis includes the following measures:

1. Cultures are made and sensitivities determined for blood, urine, all available drainage, and all possible sites of infection (eg, IV catheters, arterial and balloon catheters, Foley catheters).

2. Broad-spectrum antibiotics are given intravenously. This route gives more predictable blood levels and a more rapid onset of action than oral administration. The high mortality and severe symptoms of septic shock do not allow for the completion of sensitivity tests before drug treatment is begun. The more rapidly the therapeutic intervention is begun, the greater is the patient's chance of survival.

Where there is no specific bacteriologic information, a combination of antimicrobials directed against gram-negative enteric organisms, anaerobes, and staphylococci has been recommended.[5] An aminoglycoside such as gentamicin (Garamycin), in combination with another drug such as chloramphenicol, has been recommended; an alternative is an aminoglycoside in combination with one of the penicillinase-resistant penicillins, such as nafcillin (Nafcil, Unipen)[12] (Table 5-5).

3. If possible, the septic focus is corrected surgically (ie, drainage of abscesses, debridement of necrotic or grossly infected tissue).

Table 5-5. Antimicrobials Commonly Used in the Treatment of Sepsis

TYPE OF SEPSIS	ANTIMICROBIAL
H. influenzae or *N. meningitidis*	An aminoglycoside A penicillinase-resistant penicillin Chloramphenicol where ampicillin-resistant *H. influenzae* is common
Abdominal sepsis	An aminoglycoside, eg, gentamicin A penicillinase-resistant penicillin, eg, clindamycin (Cleocin) or chloramphenicol
Sepsis in immunodeficient patients, most commonly due to normal inhabitants of the GI tract	Carbenicillin (Geopen) in high doses, eg, 2-3 g every 2 hr Gentamicin If evidence of staphylococcal infection, a penicillinase-resistant penicillin instead of carbenicillin

4. The restoration of an adequate intravascular fluid volume is a major consideration in therapy. If the hematocrit is low, whole blood or packed cells may be given to restore volume and improve the blood's oxygen-carrying capacity. If volume expansion alone is desired, balanced salt or protein solutions are recommended. In any case, careful measurement of central venous and pulmonary artery pressures is essential to monitor fluid volume and the heart's capacity to accept fluids.

5. Because elevated body temperatures increase oxygen requirements, cooling measures are instituted for temperatures above 102°F (38.5°C).

6. Measures to improve perfusion may spontaneously correct mild metabolic acidosis by breaking the hy-

poxia-acidosis sequence. Severe acidosis worsens the prognosis because of its harmful effects on the cell; it should be treated with infusions of bicarbonate guided by the careful monitoring of laboratory values.

7. As hypoxia is the basic cause of acidosis, cell dysfunction, and death, vigorous efforts must be made to maintain a PaO_2 of at least 80 mm Hg. Endotracheal intubation with a mechanical ventilator and the use of positive end-expiratory pressure (PEEP) can be helpful in achieving adequate ventilation and preventing adult respiratory distress syndrome, which often occurs as a consequence of shock of any type.

8. Finally, massive doses of steroids may be of use. Their role in the treatment of shock is still controversial; however, proponents suggest that steroids will improve cardiac function and capillary perfusion while also reducing capillary permeability, preventing platelet aggregation, increasing oxygen availability and uptake by the cells, and stabilizing lysosomal and other membranes. The studies of Schumer[13] indicate a 42.5% mortality in patients who were not given steroids as compared with 14% in those who were. Gastrointestinal bleeding, a serious complication of steroid treatment, occurred in 3% of those studied. The incidence of gastrointestinal bleeding in septic patients not treated with steroids is almost identical.

Nursing measures

In addition to early and effective medical management, specific nursing measures are essential to the early detection and treatment of septic shock. They include the following:

1. Monitor vital signs carefully and frequently so as to detect subtle changes that occur in the early, hyperdynamic phase. Accurate baseline evaluations of respiratory rate and rhythm are necessary to detect sudden changes that may herald the onset of sepsis. For exam-

ple, even though a respiratory rate of 18 breaths per minute is considered within the normal range, it signals trouble if the patient's previous rate was 10. Also, normal breathing is almost unnoticeable; if breathing efforts are visible, the patient may have twice the normal minute ventilation.

2. Watch for such signs of impaired tissue oxygenation as changes in mental status or emotional affect, restlessness, or inappropriate behavior.

3. Look for such signs of hypovolemia as oliguria, tachycardia, thirst, dry tongue, and soft eyeballs. Also, record intake/output, including fluid losses through sweating, hyperventilation, and defecation.

4. Watch for signs of paralytic ileus as evidenced by abdominal distention and/or absent bowel sounds. Frequent checks of abdominal girth are essential to plot progressive distention accurately. Also, check stools and nasogastric aspirate for occult blood.

5. Evaluate the effectiveness of cooling measures for fever. The shivering that may accompany cooling with a hypothermia unit may actually produce more tissue hypoxia through increased metabolic demand. A drug that diminishes shivering, such as chlorpromazine (Thorazine), may be given for more efficient cooling.

6. Make sure that oxygen administration equipment remains properly positioned, so that the patient derives optimal benefit from oxygen therapy.

7. Administer all medications as quickly as possible, since the outcome in shock depends largely on speedy intervention. Also, be aware of possible drug reactions and interactions.

8. Make sure that all specimens for laboratory work are obtained quickly and accurately.

9. Allow the patient time to rest. Dirty linen, for example, produces no adverse physiologic effects; however, moving the unstable patient for baths or changes of linen may well do so.

REFERENCES

1. Hinshaw LB: Overview of endotoxin shock. In *Pathophysiology of Shock, Anoxia, and Ischemia* (Cowley RA, Trump BF, eds), pp 219-235. Baltimore: Williams & Wilkins, 1982

2. McCabe WR: Gram negative bacteremia. *Adv Intern Med* 19:135, 1974

3. Bryan-Brown C, Christy JD, Fearnon DT, et al: *Septic Shock.* Kalamazoo, Mi: The Upjohn Company, 1977

4. Shatney CH, Dietzman RH, Lillehei RC: Effects of early administration of corticosteroids in clinical septic shock. In *3rd International Symposium in Critical Care Medicine*, Rio de Janeiro, 1974, p 71

5. Weil MH: Bacteremic (septic) shock: Diagnosis and management. In *Summary Proceedings of the Twentieth Annual Symposium on Critical Care Medicine,* p 65. University of Southern California School of Medicine, Postgraduate Division, Las Vegas, 1982

6. Thomas L: *The Lives of a Cell.* New York: Viking, 1974

7. Robinson JA, Klodyncky ML, Loeb HS, et al: Endotoxin, prekallikrein, complement and systemic vascular resistance. *Am J Med* 59:61, 1975

8. Winslow EJ, Loeb HS, Rahimtoola SH, et al: Hemodynamic studies and results of therapy in fifty patients with bacteremic shock. *Am J Med* 54:421, 1973

9. Ayres SM, Giannelle S, Mueller HS, Peuhler ME: *Care of the Critically Ill,* 2nd ed, p 282. New York: Appleton-Century-Crofts, 1974

10. Jacob HS: *Role of Complement and Granulocytes in Septic Shock.* Rahway, NJ: The Upjohn Company, 1978

11. Virgilio RW, Smith DE: Assessment and therapy of the shock syndrome. *Emergency Care, Assessment and Intervention* (Spraule, Mullanney, eds). St. Louis: Mosby, 1974

12. Gardner P, Provine H: *Manual of Acute Bacterial Infections,* pp 155-164. Boston: Little, Brown, 1980

13. Schumer W: Steroids in the treatment of clinical septic shock. *Ann Surg* 184:33, 1976

6

CARDIOGENIC SHOCK

BILLIE C. MEADOR, RN, MS, CCRN

Cardiogenic shock, as its name implies, is caused by abnormal functioning of the heart, specifically the ventricles, which fail to pump properly. This, in turn, may stem from various causes—tension pneumothorax, pericardial tamponade, pulmonary embolism, disturbances in heart rate or rhythm, heart disease, myocardial infarction, drug reactions, and others. The symptoms are similar to those of hypovolemic shock, discussed in Chapter 4. The difference is simply that in hypovolemic shock there is not enough intravascular fluid to be pumped, whereas in cardiogenic shock the pump itself is not working as it should. The result is that, as in all other forms of shock, the body's cells are deprived of the oxygen and nutrients they need to sustain life (see Chapter 1).

Most commonly, cardiogenic shock arises from myocardial infarction; about 15 to 20% of such patients experience it. Its presence indicates that at least 40% of the myocardial muscle mass has been damaged or destroyed, and it is associated with a very high mortality (between 80 and 100%). There are signs that this rate is on the decline. If that is true, it is surely because treatment techniques have improved as the mechanisms of shock have come to be more clearly understood. In the case of cardiogenic shock, the use of drugs has proved especially helpful. These are discussed under "Pharmacology in cardiogenic shock," below.

Diagnosis

Myocardial infarction

Myocardial infarction is the most frequent cause of cardiogenic shock. Clinical signs and symptoms of MI include chest pain, nausea and vomiting, shortness of breath, hypotension, rales, sweating, pallor, weakness, tachycardia, fever, and elevated white blood count.

However, the diagnosis is confirmed by laboratory tests and ECG analysis.

Enzymes. Three enzymes—creatine kinase, lactate dehydrogenase, and aspartate aminotransferase—are generally used to test for MI. "Normal" values vary from laboratory to laboratory, so determine what is considered normal in your institution. Patterns, rather than specific numbers, are important. All of these enzymes are usually found intracellularly. Although small amounts are normally found in the serum, large amounts mean damage to or destruction of cells, causing their enzymes to be liberated into the serum.

Creatine kinase (CK), formerly called creatine phosphokinase (CPK), is normally found in the tissues of the heart, brain, and skeletal muscles. Anything that stresses the heart (infarction, failure, defibrillation, pulmonary embolism) or skeletal muscles (exercise, repeated intramuscular injections) may elevate CK levels; elevations due to brain disorders are less common. When an elevated CK is reported, it is impossible to tell which area it comes from without analyzing isoenzymes. There are three isoenzymes of CK, found in the different tissues (Table 6-1). An elevated CK_2 (MB bands) is present in

Table 6-1. Isoenzymes of Creatine Kinase and Lactate Dehydrogenase

ISOENZYME	COMPOSITION	TISSUE
CK_1	BB	Brain
CK_2	MB	Myocardium
CK_3	MM	Skeletal muscle
LDH_1	HHHH	Mostly cardiac
LDH_2	HHHM	Mostly cardiac
LDH_3	HHMM	Largely pulmonary
LDH_4	HMMM	Mostly used for liver disease
LDH_5	MMMM	Mostly used for liver disease

Table 6-2. Patterns of Enzyme Change in Myocardial Infarction

ENZYME	"NORMAL" VALUE (IU/LITER)	FIRST RISES (HOURS)	PEAKS (HOURS)
CK	50-230	3-4	33
LDH	36-200	12-24	72
SGOT	8-30	6-8	24-48

almost all MIs, but is not an infallible indicator of MI. Nor is it known what level of CK_2 is significant.

A total lactate dehydrogenase (LDH) is not much more useful than a total CK. However, LDH can also be fractionated, or broken down, into isoenzymes (Table 6-1). Normally, the ratio of LDH_1 to LDH_2 is less than 1:1. When the level of LDH_1 rises to a point where the ratio exceeds 1:1 (becomes "flipped") following a significant elevation of CK_2, most clinicians consider it diagnostic of an infarct.

Aspartate aminotransferase (SGOT, formerly serum glutamic-oxaloacetic transaminase) is found in many areas of the body. It has no isoenzyme and is used primarily in liver disease.

Table 6-2 summarizes the patterns of change of these enzymes in MI and also lists their "normal" values.

Electrocardiographic changes. The ECG changes that are diagnostic of an infarct are complicated and are beyond the scope of the book. However, three general types of changes are seen:

- T-wave inversions indicate ischemia.
- ST elevations indicate injury.
- Q waves indicate necrosis.

All these changes are indicative of damage. Determination of the location of the damage is based on which leads these changes appear in (Table 6-3).

Table 6-3. Correlation Between ECG Leads and Location of Cardiac Damage

LEAD	LOCATION OF DAMAGE
V_1	Anterior, posterior
V_2	Anterior, posterior
V_3	Anterior, septal
V_4	Septal
V_5	Lateral
V_6	Lateral
I	Lateral
II	Inferior
III	Inferior
AVF	Inferior
AVL	Lateral
AVR	Lateral

Cardiogenic shock

To determine the severity of cardiogenic shock, the arteriovenous oxygen difference (a-vDO_2), or oxygen debt, is measured (see Chapter 3). An a-vDO_2 of 6 vol% or more indicates that cardiac decompensation is present; that is, the heart has been damaged so severely that cardiac output is no longer adequate for tissue perfusion.

Other signs and symptoms include the following:[1-3]

1. Systolic blood pressure either below 90 mm Hg or at least 30 mm Hg (or more) below the patient's normal pressure
2. Decreased mentation (due to decreased perfusion to the cerebral tissues)
3. Oliguria—less than 20 to 25 mL/h (due to decreased perfusion to the kidneys as well as the natural tendency of the kidneys to retain fluid in the presence of decreased renal perfusion)
4. Tachycardia
5. Cold, clammy skin
6. S_3 or S_4 or both
7. Arrhythmia

8. Hyperventilation
9. Mottling of the extremities, particularly the legs, as peripheral perfusion is compromised
10. Other symptoms relating to the etiology of the shock or preexisting pathology.

Assessment of the patient in shock is covered in greater detail in Chapter 2.

Goals of therapy

Overall goals of therapy in cardiogenic shock are to:

1. Increase myocardial oxygenation while decreasing utilization
2. Decrease metabolic acidosis
3. Stimulate the strength of myocardial contraction
4. Prevent secondary, potentially fatal insults such as adult respiratory distress syndrome, acute renal failure, or mesenteric infarction.

Treatment

The following measures are intended to achieve the goals outlined above:

1. Administration of supplemental oxygen
2. Stabilization of cardiac function
3. Intravenous analgesia (morphine) if indicated (subcutaneous or intramuscular administration must be *avoided* since there is poor tissue perfusion and erratic uptake)
4. Hourly measurement of urinary output
5. Frequent arterial blood gas measurements to monitor acidosis and aid in its treatment
6. Cardiac output measurements to evaluate the progress of the shock and the effectiveness of the therapy

7. Support of blood pressure through the use of drugs such as dobutamine (Dobutrex) and dopamine (Intropin)
8. Suppression of arrhythmias
9. Hemodynamic monitoring (discussed under "Pharmacology," below; see also Chapter 3, "Monitoring the Patient in Shock").

The intraaortic balloon or counterpulsation device may also be used in treating the patient. This balloon is usually inserted in the operating room by a cardiothoracic surgeon. However, newer forms of this device allow it to be inserted percutaneously. It is threaded retrograde through the femoral artery into the aorta. The balloon is then positioned so that its proximal end is below the bifurcation of the subclavian artery and the distal end is above the bifurcation of the renal arteries. The balloon is then attached to the machine, which coordinates its actions with the electrocardiograph. It is designed to deflate during systole, thus decreasing the work of the heart by decreasing afterload. As it inflates during diastole, it increases perfusion pressure, which results in greater blood flow to the tissues and the coronary arteries. This useful therapy has many potentially lethal complications and should be used only by skilled practitioners. Refer to supplemental resources for more detailed information on this piece of equipment.[4-6]

Pharmacology in cardiogenic shock

In treating this form of shock, medications may be used extensively. They are given in order to achieve four major goals:

1. To decrease afterload
2. To alter preload
3. To increase contractility
4. To increase peripheral perfusion.

Decreasing afterload

Afterload is the resistance that must be overcome in order to eject the stroke volume. Aortic stenosis and systemic hypertension are two examples of conditions that increase afterload. The condition most commonly seen in cardiogenic shock is peripheral vasoconstriction, a result of sympathetic stimulation.

Two drugs, sodium nitroprusside (Nipride) and nitroglycerin, are used to decrease afterload. The choice between them depends on the physician's preference.

Sodium nitroprusside is given intravenously, usually in concentrations of 50 mg/100 mL 5% dextrose in water, though other strengths may be used. Sodium nitroprusside is incompatible with normal saline. Once mixed, the solution is stable for 24 hours and must be protected from direct light. The therapeutic dose is 0.5 to 10 μg/kg/min. It is imperative that the person who is administering the drug be aware of the dose in terms of micrograms per kilogram per minute and not drops per minute. Given the same concentration and drip rate, the actual delivered dose will vary with patients of different body weights. Sodium nitroprusside is metabolized into thiocyanate cyanide ion and can produce cyanide poisoning. Serum thiocyanate or cyanide levels must be monitored daily in any patient receiving the drug either in high doses or for prolonged periods.[7, 8]

Intravenous nitroglycerin is an alternative to nitroprusside that is gaining increasing acceptance because its effects are easier to control, although it is not as effective a peripheral vasodilator. It is usually mixed in a glass bottle in a concentration of 25 to 200 mg in 100 to 500 mL of 5% dextrose in water or normal saline. The dose is measured in milligrams per kilogram per minute and is titrated according to the patient's response and the severity of side effects: headache, nausea and vomiting, tachycardia, restlessness, and hypotension.

Altering preload

Preload is the end-diastolic volume or pressure, and adequate filling pressure is necessary for the ventricles to pump sufficient stroke volume and therefore cardiac output. Preload is monitored using the pulmonary capillary wedge pressure. When there is excess volume, the ventricular fibers are stretched beyond the physiological limits of Starling's law; the result is a less than optimal contraction. In this case diuretics are indicated to help decrease the circulating volume. (Also see "Increasing contractility," below.) Furosemide (Lasix) is usually used because of its rapid onset and potency.

Starling's law implies that the ventricles can pump out only what they receive. A decrease in circulating volume means that there is insufficient venous return to allow an adequate stroke volume and cardiac output. Therefore, in cases of decreased volume, volume replacement is indicated. A fluid challenge such as 200 mL of normal saline, 5% dextrose solution, or plasma protein fraction (Plasmanate) over 15 minutes may be given to evaluate the effectiveness of volume replacement. Further replacement may be done with crystalloids or colloids, depending on the severity of the depletion and the physician's preference.

Increasing contractility

Contractility is the pumping force of the ventricles. Increases in contractility result in increases in stroke volume, provided that there is adequate circulating volume. The effects of increasing ventricular contractility are seen by monitoring the cardiac output. Three drugs may be used, alone or in combination: digoxin (Lanoxin), dopamine, and dobutamine.

While it increases contractility, digoxin also provides a direct and indirect decrease in heart rate. Its uses and actions are well known and need not be discussed further here.

To increase contractility, dopamine is given in doses of approximately 5 to 15 μg/kg/min. Lower doses have little cardiac effect (see "Increasing peripheral perfusion," below) and higher doses produce peripheral vasoconstriction, thus increasing afterload. The dose must be given in micrograms per kilogram per minute, not in drops per minute, in order to obtain the desired effects. Dopamine may increase the heart rate and cause ventricular irritability, but these effects are rarely so great as to call for an alteration of dosage. The drug is incompatible with alkaline solutions.[7, 8]

Dobutamine is pharmacologically similar to dopamine. In contrast to dopamine, however, dobutamine is specifically indicated for short-term use. Dobutamine does not have dopamine's advantage of increasing mesenteric and renal blood flow. Dobutamine may also cause an increase in heart rate and ventricular irritability. The usual dose is 2.5 to 20 μg/kg/min. Like dopamine, this drug is incompatible with alkaline solutions.

Increasing peripheral perfusion

Peripheral perfusion is very important in shock of any kind. Inadequate peripheral perfusion results in anaerobic metabolism, elevations in lactic acid, and metabolic acidosis. Perfusion may be compromised to the point of inducing failure of organ systems. The kidneys and the mesentery are especially vulnerable. Adequate peripheral perfusion is accomplished through vasodilation. Sodium nitroprusside provides general vasodilation to all areas. Dopamine, in doses of less than 5 to 7 μg/kg/min, provides vasodilation specifically to the mesentery and the kidneys. These two drugs are frequently used in combination. It is important to remember that adequate peripheral perfusion is not possible without an adequate circulating volume. Therefore, any deficit in this regard should be corrected without delay.[7, 8]

REFERENCES

1. Pice SA, Wilson LM: *Pathophysiology: Clinical Concepts of Disease Processes.* New York: McGraw-Hill, 1982

2. Sodeman WA, Sodeman TM: *Pathologic Physiology: Mechanisms of Disease,* 5th ed. Philadelphia: Saunders, 1974

3. Kinney MR: *AACN's Clinical Reference for Critical-Care Nursing.* New York: McGraw-Hill, 1981

4. Bulls S: Intra-aortic balloon pump. *Crit Care Update* p 5, September 1976

5. Dorr KS: The intra-aortic balloon pump. *Crit Care Update* p 12, February 1978

6. Eckhardt E: Intra-aortic balloon counterpulsation in cardiogenic shock. *Heart Lung* 6:93, 1977

7. Shinn A: The current use of dopamine and nitroprusside. *Crit Care Update* p 28, August 1978

8. Shearer J, Caldwell M: Use of sodium nitroprusside and dopamine hydrochloride in the postoperative cardiac patient. *Heart Lung* 8:302, 1979

7

NEUROGENIC SHOCK

LUANNE M. FRANCO, RN, MSN, CCRN

The clinical syndrome of shock in relation to the central nervous system may be considered from the viewpoints of both causes and effects. This chapter will deal with the causes of neurogenic shock, especially spinal shock, and the effects of shock in general on the central nervous system.

Pathophysiology

Neurogenic shock is essentially shock initiated through the action (or inaction) of the central nervous system. Like the other shock syndromes already discussed (see Chapters 4, 5, and 6), it involves massive vasodilation, decreased peripheral vascular resistance, and increased vascular capacity. The pathophysiology, in short, is not markedly different from that already outlined, especially in Chapters 1 and 2.

Signs and symptoms

The clinical picture of neurogenic shock differs from that of classic hypovolemic shock in that the blood pressure may be extremely low, with a decrease in the pulse rate. The skin is usually dry, warm, and flushed. Urine output is frequently within normal limits. Finally, there is a definite neurologic deficit in neurogenic shock, whereas this is usually not the case in the early stages of hypovolemic shock.

Etiology

Neurogenic shock can be caused by any of the following events: exposure to unpleasant circumstances (eg, fright), pain, high spinal anesthesia, spinal cord injury, vasomotor depression, and head injury.

Neurogenic shock may be manifested clinically as syncope after exposure to an unpleasant sight or a frightening stimulus. Such stimuli have been found to increase vagal stimulation of the heart, causing bradycardia and decreased cardiac output along with peripheral vasodilation. When an individual faints and falls to a horizontal position, normal cardiac output is reinstituted almost immediately and the person soon recovers fully. If, however, this individual were to be kept in an upright position (for example, by being crushed in a throng), the shock cycle would be perpetuated by the fall in cardiac output; irreversible shock might then ensue.

Although transient hypotension may occur after head injury, sustained hypotension in the head-injured patient is almost always due to causes outside the cranium. The exception is overwhelming, eventually fatal cerebral injury in adults, where hypotension is caused by injury to the vasomotor center in the medulla. Then it is not unusual to see wide fluctuations in blood pressure, ranging from severe hypotension to severe hypertension.

Injuries to the spinal cord or interruption of its function can also lead to neurogenic shock. During high spinal anesthesia or after transection of the spinal cord above T-6, shock can develop from the interruption of sympathetic impulses traveling from the vasomotor center of the medulla to the peripheral blood vessels. Since these sympathetic impulses govern vasoconstriction, generalized vasodilation is produced.

The treatment of neurogenic shock caused by high spinal anesthesia includes the administration of ephedrine or phenylephrine. These drugs increase cardiac output and cause peripheral vasoconstriction.

Spinal shock

In the United States, the incidence of spinal cord injury is approximately 50 cases per million people per year.[1]

The clinical picture of spinal cord injury is often compounded by the syndrome of spinal shock. Approximately 30 to 60 minutes after injury, edema of the spinal cord develops and causes a physiologic transection of spinal cord function. Spinal shock, a transient depression of spinal function below the level of injury, then sets in and causes a number of physiologic sequelae: hypotension, bradycardia, disturbances of temperature regulation, paralytic ileus, and transient urinary and fecal retention. The period of spinal shock persists for 1 to 6 weeks; recovery from the effects of spinal shock can take from 6 to 12 months.[2]

Cardiovascular effects

Cardiovascular responses may be triggered when a sudden, traumatic spinal cord transection initiates spinal shock. Sympathetic nervous system outflow occurs between T-1 and L-2 and is responsible for vasoconstriction as well as for increased heart rate and myocardial contractility.

Impairment of the sympathetic nervous system

In spinal cord injuries that transect the cord at the level of T-6 or above, the sympathetic nervous system is severely impaired. One effect is hypotension, caused by the blockage of vasoconstrictive impulses. This not only lowers the blood pressure but also causes pooling of blood in the peripheral circulation, which leads to a decreased venous return to the heart and a decrease in cardiac output. The loss of the vasoconstrictive property of blood vessels may have serious consequences in a patient with multisystem injury. In shock caused by hypovolemia, the body employs vasoconstriction as a protective compensatory mechanism to maintain adequate perfusion pressure to the vital body organs. A patient suffering from spinal shock has lost the ability to compensate by vasoconstriction and may progress rapidly into an irreversible shock state.

Blood pressure changes

In the patient with spinal shock alone, the blood pressure will usually stabilize at 100/60 mm Hg. If this stabilization takes place, urine output remains between 30 and 40 mL/h, and the patient shows no change in mental status, no corrective measures are necessary. However, if the mean systemic arterial pressure falls below 70 mm Hg, fluid replacement is required and should be employed with the help of a central venous pressure monitor so as to prevent fluid overload. In this instance, other causes of hypotension must be investigated.

Disturbed cardiac rate and rhythm

Another cardiovascular effect of spinal shock is a disturbance of cardiac rate and rhythm. Cardioacceleratory responses mediated by the sympathetic nervous system are blocked, allowing cardioinhibitory impulses to predominate. In previously healthy individuals, it is unnecessary to treat a sinus bradycardia unless the heart rate falls below 40 beats per minute. Patients with a severe bradycardia may need to be given an anticholinergic such as atropine. In cases of severe bradycardia with sinus arrest, a temporary transvenous pacemaker may be inserted.

Vagal impulses to the sinoatrial node are unopposed in spinal shock, so it is important to minimize vagal stimulation (Valsalva maneuver, tracheal suctioning) in these patients. In the case of tracheal suctioning, adequate oxygenation before and after should minimize the vagal response.

Fluctuations in body temperature

The patient suffering from spinal shock may also show a disturbance in body temperature control. The sympathetic pathway leading from the hypothalamic temperature control center to the blood vessels is disrupted. This pathway regulates vasodilation and sweating when the temperature of the environment rises, and vasoconstriction and shivering when the environmental temperature falls. Thus, the patient with spinal shock may become poikilothermic, that is, the body temperature will fluctuate in response to changes in the surrounding temperature. If the room becomes too warm, the patient's body temperature will rise; if the room temperature falls, so will the patient's body temperature.

Special care must be taken to keep the temperature of the patient's environment as moderate and as constant as possible, since the patient has no control over the body's temperature. A constantly fluctuating temperature carries a risk of hyperthermia, which will increase metabolic demands for oxygen, or hypothermia, which predisposes the patient to the development of life-threatening dysrhythmias.

Disruption of gastrointestinal or urinary system

In addition to cardiovascular complications, a patient with spinal shock may show disruptions of the gastrointestinal or genitourinary system. With spinal cord injury, peristalsis ceases within 24 hours after the moment of injury and does not resume for approximately 3 to 4 days. Gastric dilation may occur, along with paralytic ileus; both are attributed to loss of central control over the digestive system.[3] Gastric dilation may cause hypoxemia by interfering with the function of the diaphragm. In addition, both gastric dilation and paralytic ileus may cause vomiting, with resultant pulmonary aspiration; this, of course, can lead to respiratory failure. Until bowel sounds return, therefore, a nasogastric tube should be inserted and connected to suction. With the removal of gastric contents, metabolic alkalosis may result from the loss of chloride and hydrogen ions along with potassium. Careful monitoring of serum electrolytes is important to prevent complications associated with electrolyte and acid-base imbalances.

After spinal cord injury, the contractile ability of the urinary bladder is lost, leading to urinary retention. This condition may persist for weeks or even months after injury. An indwelling catheter is inserted initially after injury so that the patient's fluid balance can be monitored closely. Intermittent catheterization is the preferred method of treatment; however, it is generally not employed until after the acute phase of injury.[4]

Nursing implications

Nursing care of the patient who is suffering from neurogenic shock involves accurate, continuous assessment, troubleshooting for complications, and prompt intervention. A baseline patient assessment is essential. This assessment comprises vital signs (including temperature) and neurologic status (including a statement describing the level of consciousness, pupil size and reaction to light, score on the Glasgow coma scale, the ability to obey commands, and strength and movement in the extremities).

Other areas of neurologic function should be tested as well, including reaction to pain, sensory impairment, and changes in reflexes. (Assessment for reaction to painful stimuli will also help to detect alterations in sensory perception.)

The pinprick test

Being sure that the patient's eyes are closed, touch him very lightly with a pin on various areas of the body. It can be useful to alternate between the sharp and dull ends of the pin, asking the patient whether there is any sensation and, if so, whether it is sharp or dull. The use of a dermatome sheet to record the patient's responses makes it possible to recognize progression or regression of the sensory alterations.

Sacral sparing

The patient with spinal cord injury should also be tested for the presence of sacral sparing, which is a good prognostic sign. (The sensory tracts of the sacral segments of the cord are located on the cord's periphery and are more resistant to injury.) In essence, sacral sparing is the preservation of sacral segmental sensation and reflex; it indicates that the cord lesion is incomplete and that there is significant chance for the recovery of some spinal cord function. The accepted test for this is the anal "wink" reflex. To provoke it, lightly stimulate the anus with the sharp end of a pin; if sacral sparing is present, the anal sphincter will contract.

Effects of shock on the brain

The clinical symptoms of neurogenic shock can affect almost every body system. You must have a working knowledge of the relevant pathophysiology so that you can troubleshoot for possible complications and act promptly to minimize their consequences.

Although the brain weighs only about 1,360 g, cerebral blood flow accounts for 15% of the cardiac output. Cerebral oxygen consumption is 3.5 mL/100 g/min, or 20% of the total oxygen consumed by the body. The brain needs large amounts of oxygen to oxidize enough glucose to meet its high metabolic demands.

In order to ensure adequate cerebral blood flow and oxygenation despite wide variations in systemic arterial pressure, the brain employs a mechanism called autoregulation, which helps to keep the cerebral perfusion pressure (CPP) steady. CPP is the pressure difference between the arterial blood entering the brain and the venous blood leaving the brain; it can be calculated by subtracting the intracranial pressure (ICP) from the mean systemic arterial pressure (MAP). Normal CPP is between 80 and 90 mm Hg. With a CPP below 60 mm Hg, cerebral blood flow begins to diminish. If the CPP drops below 50 mm Hg, there is neuronal dysfunction; below 30 mm Hg, neuronal death occurs. Cerebral blood flow ceases when the ICP equals the CPP.

During shock, temporary global brain ischemia generally develops. This is simply another way of saying underperfusion. Although the brain's autoregulatory mechanism will cause cerebral vasodilation in an attempt to maintain adequate cerebral blood flow, this compensatory mechanism lasts only until the MAP drops to 50 mm Hg. Below this level the patient is likely to experience a decreased level of consciousness. If the MAP drops below 30 mm Hg and the cerebral blood flow is less than 20% of normal, the pupils will dilate and the neurons will die.

As the brain cells undergo anaerobic metabolism, the production of ATP decreases and lactic acid builds up. Sodium and water move into the cells; potassium exits. The cells swell and ultimately rupture, spilling their contents into the cerebral circulation. These cellular contents, or "injury agents," are lysosomal enzymes that can be toxic to cerebral tissue.

Clinically, the patient in neurogenic shock may exhibit focal neurologic deficits, confusion, stupor, or coma. Specific clinical signs will depend on the area of the brain involved. For example, if the hypothalamus suffers ischemia, the body's normal temperature-regulating mechanism will be disrupted and the patient will experience both hyperthermia and hypothermia. Brain stem ischemia may damage the reticular activating system, causing stupor or coma. Again, specific clinical symptoms will depend on the area of the brain that is affected. It is therefore imperative to have a thorough basic understanding of neuroanatomy and physiology so that you can correlate clinical symptoms with the underlying pathophysiology.

In summary, neurogenic shock may be seen from two points of view: its origin within the nervous system and also its effects upon it. Since these effects are extremely dangerous and often irreversible, intelligent nursing of these patients can help to preserve quality of life as well as life itself.

REFERENCES

1. Kraus JF: Injury to the head and the spinal cord. The epidemiological relevance of the medical literature published from 1960 to 1980. *J Neurosurg* suppl S3, 1980

2. Davis J, Mason CB: *Neurologic Critical Care.* New York: Van Nostrand Reinhold, 1978

3. Guttman L: Spinal shock. In *Handbook of Clinical Neurology* (Vinken PJ, Bruyn GW, eds). New York: American Elsevier, 1976.

4. Donovan WH, Bedbrook G: *Comprehensive Management of Spinal Cord Injuries.* Ciba Clinical Symposia, vol 34, 1982

8

ANAPHYLACTIC SHOCK

GLORIA SONNESSO, RN, MSN, CCRN

Case study

K. D., a 21-year-old white woman, had been diagnosed with histiocytosis X and diabetes insipidus. She was admitted to the hospital complaining of increasing shortness of breath over approximately a week, and muscular aches and diarrhea for approximately 2 weeks prior to admission. Her past medical history was unremarkable. She had a known allergy to penicillin and had had one childhood reaction to a bee sting, which was treated in an emergency room.

At this admission, her vital signs were as follows: temperature, 96.6°F; heart rate, 85; blood pressure, 90/50; and respiratory rate, 24. Four days after admission, a bronchoscopy was performed. She was medicated with 1.5 mg of hydromorphone hydrochloride (Dilaudid) and 0.6 mg of atropine and tolerated the procedure well.

Approximately 30 minutes after the bronchoscopy, she complained of increasing shortness of breath and had both peripheral cyanosis and short, shallow, rapid respirations. She was given one ampoule of naloxone hydrochloride (Narcan) IV to counteract the hydromorphone but did not improve. The patient became tachycardic and hypotensive. At this time, IV administration of 1,000 mL of normal saline was started at a wide-open drip. Arterial blood gases were found to be as follows: pH, 7.23; pCO_2, 53; and pO_2, 30—indicating acidosis. She was to be transferred out of the medical surgical unit to the respiratory ICU when she suffered cardiac arrest. The code team was called and successful resuscitation performed. Still intubated with the endotracheal tube used in the code, and with manual ventilation, she was transferred to the respiratory ICU. At that time her arterial blood gases were: pH, 7.02; pO_2, 23.

Dopamine (Intropin) was started IV immediately after her arrival in the respiratory unit. Despite the continuing wide-open drip, her blood pressure remained in the hypotensive range. Central venous and arterial lines were inserted and plans made to insert a pulmonary artery line as soon as her condition stabilized.

A stat portable chest x-ray showed pulmonary edema. She was therefore placed on an MA-II ventilator with an FiO_2 of 100% and 10 cm PEEP. She was given three doses of epinephrine (Adrenalin) and 1 g of methylprednisolone sodium succinate (Solu-Medrol).

One hour after her first crisis, despite the treatment and medications, she still had refractory hypotension and increasing bradycardia. An isoproterenol (Isuprel) drip was started, followed by an epinephrine drip, but the hypotension and bradycardia persisted.

A short time later, a repeat chest x-ray revealed a pneumomediastinum and a right pneumothorax. Chest tubes were inserted into the right and left sides to remove the air and reinflate the lung. At this time, it was suspected that a cardiac tamponade might be causing the hypotension and bradycardia. A pericardial tap was performed and 100 mL of clear fluid were aspirated.

Despite continued efforts to save her, the patient was pronounced dead 2½ hours after the bronchoscopy was completed. What caused this young, stable, essentially healthy young woman to die? Several answers were possible. An allergy to hydromorphone hydrochloride was ruled out because of the time that passed between its administration and the onset of symptoms. At autopsy, the diagnosis was death due to anaphylactic shock. The causative agent: lidocaine (Xylocaine), used during the bronchoscopy.

Etiology

Anaphylaxis is a potentially lethal reaction to some precipitating antigen that can occur within minutes of exposure. The precipitating antigen may originate from insect venom, a drug, or dye used in radiological studies. The reaction can be local or systemic; and often, a local reaction will precede a systemic one.

Signs and symptoms

The first signs of a reaction are a vague uneasiness, dizziness, and nausea. If the cause is a bee sting or insect bite, there may be local redness, itching, and swelling. More severe reactions lead to generalized body itching, hives, hot skin, and diffuse erythema. There can be rapid progression to stridor, dysphagia, and dyspnea, angioedema of the face, hands, and feet, and bronchospasm, laryngeal edema, and respiratory arrest with concurrent cardiovascular collapse.

Pathogenesis

The anaphylactic mechanism is thought to be twofold:
1. When the antigen is first introduced into the body, a specific IGE antibody is formed, which then binds to mast cells and basophils.
2. When exposure to the antigen is repeated, a response by the IGE antibodies is triggered, resulting in the release of three chemical mediators: histamine, slow-reacting substance of anaphylaxis (SRS-A), and bradykinin.

Histamine acts to dilate arterioles, capillaries, and venules and increases their cell wall permeability. It also causes contraction of nonvascular smooth muscle, leading to bronchospasm.

SRS-A, a lipid substance, also affects nonvascular smooth muscle, causing intense bronchoconstriction, and vascular smooth muscle, causing dilation and increasing the permeability of the venules' cell walls.

Bradykinin, a peptide substance, works similarly, causing vasodilation, increased capillary permeability, and bronchoconstriction.

These substances have profound effects on the pulmonary and vascular systems. A person having an *acute* anaphylactic reaction will have severe bronchospasm and laryngeal edema, requiring intubation and perhaps even an emergency tracheostomy to maintain a patent airway. There will be profound hypotension due to volume loss and tachycardia, along with loss of consciousness and a markedly decreased urine output.

Treatment

If the victim is to survive an anaphylactic reaction, it must be recognized and treated within minutes. Minor local reactions can be treated with ice—to cause vasoconstriction and inhibit spread—and antihistamines. Diphenhydramine hydrochloride (Benadryl) is the most commonly used antihistamine; it is given in doses of 25 to 50 mg IM or IV. In more severe local reactions, epinephrine 0.2 to 0.5 mg may be given subcutaneously.

More acute anaphylactic reactions must be treated aggressively. If a medication (eg, a drug or dye) is thought to be the cause of the reaction, it must be discontinued immediately. The airway must be guaranteed by either intubation or tracheostomy. Epinephrine 0.2 to 0.5 mg IV or IM is given immediately. The major effort then is to support the patient hemodynamically until the anaphylactic reaction is controlled. Careful monitoring is essential, especially of vital signs and fluid balance. Volume replacement with crystalloids and colloids is done to replace the fluid lost through leakage from the capillaries and to compensate for the profound vasodilation. Pressor agents (eg, dopamine, norepinephrine, or isoproterenol) may be given IV. High doses of corticosteroids are given to decrease capillary permeability—thereby maintaining volume—and to stabilize the mast cells so as to prevent the further release of chemical mediators. If treatment is initiated in a timely fashion, there will be few or no side effects.

The nurse's role

The nurse's role in anaphylaxis is twofold. First, of course, you must be able to recognize possible anaphylaxis and know how to assist in its emergency treatment. Second, and more important, is your role in preventing the development of these reactions by taking a detailed nursing history from the patient or family and informing all those personnel involved in the patient's care of any possible allergies.

Thorough questioning of the patient about reactions to food or medication he's experienced in the past can be very valuable in preventing an anaphylactic reaction. Food allergies often indicate a potential allergy to medication; for example, an allergy to shellfish may indicate sensitivity to iodine-containing dyes, or an allergy to eggs may precipitate a reaction to flu vaccine, which is often derived from chick embryos.

Once the history is complete, you can play an important role in helping to educate the patient about the importance of allergies—being aware of them and not being afraid to inform people about them. Warn patients to check the contents of over-the-counter medications carefully and never to take anyone else's medications, since they may contain some substance to which the patient is allergic.

A patient with allergies should be advised to wear a Medic-Alert bracelet or tag, which, in the event of an emergency, will inform health care personnel of a possible problem.

In a time when new medications for treatment and diagnosis are constantly being developed, it is the nurse's responsibility to be aware of the potential for anaphylactic reactions and aid in their prevention.

GENERAL REFERENCES

Beeson PB, McDermott W, Wyngaarden JB: *Cecil Textbook of Medicine,* 15th ed. Philadelphia: Saunders, 1979

Furth R: Anaphylaxis and drug reactions: Guidelines for detection and care. *Heart Lung* 9:662, 1980

Guyton AC: *Textbook of Medical Physiology,* 3rd ed. Philadelphia: Saunders, 1970

Harmon AL, Harmon DC: Anaphylaxis—Sudden death anytime. *Nursing 80* 10(10):40, October 1980

Meyers FH, Jawetz E, Goldfien A: *Review of Medical Pharmacology,* 7th ed. Los Altos, Calif: Lange, 1980

9

DISSEMINATED INTRAVASCULAR COAGULATION

PATRICIA A. MEEHAN, RN, MS, CCRN

Disseminated intravascular coagulopathy is one of the life-threatening complications of shock. It has many synonyms, including defibrination syndrome, consumptive coagulopathy, and intravascular thrombosis; the most common is simply DIC.[1] This phenomenon comprises a sequence of events resulting from the abnormal, diffuse activation of coagulation and fibrinolysis. It is both a bleeding disease and a thrombotic disorder[1] (Figure 9-1). DIC has the effect of converting the circulating plasma into serum and is an extremely serious, often terminal condition.

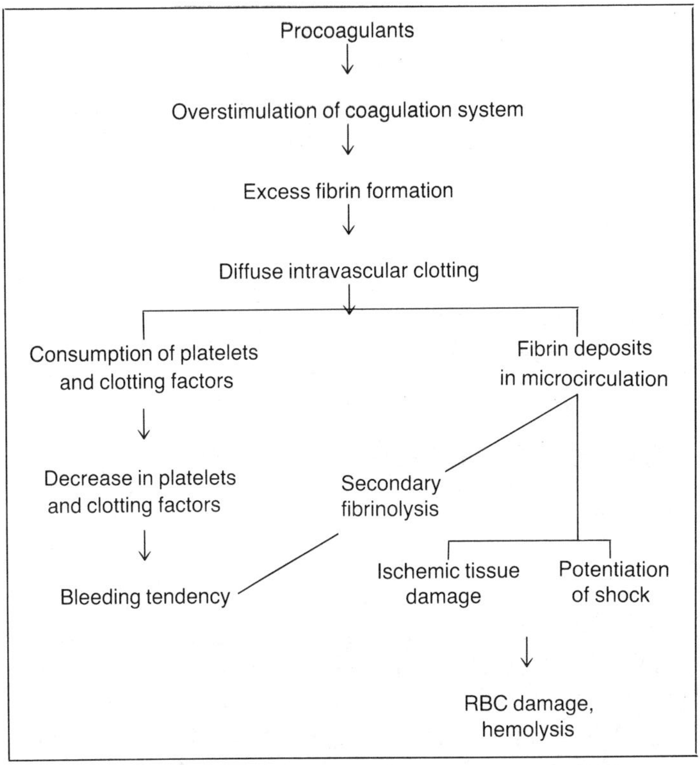

Figure 9-1. The mechanism of DIC. Adapted from Williams WJ, et al: Hematology, p 1235. New York: McGraw-Hill, 1972; and O'Brian B, Woods S: Paradox of DIC. Am J Nurs 78:1878, 1978.

The mechanism of DIC

DIC occurs when procoagulants (eg, platelets, calcium ions, thromboplastin, bacterial endotoxins, certain lipid substances) activate the coagulation system and normal defense mechanisms malfunction.[2] Overstimulation of the coagulation process leads to the formation of excess fibrin, causing small thrombi to develop in the microcirculation.[3] Ischemic tissue damage and red blood cell hemolysis may occur as a result. The widespread clotting causes thrombocytopenia, because platelets are caught up in the increasing number of aggregates. A shortage of plasma clotting factors I, II, V, VIII (see Table 9-1) develops because they are consumed more rapidly than they can be replenished. Rapid secondary activation of the fibrinolytic system produces fibrinogen degradation products (FDPs) and causes a marked reduction in serum fibrinogen.[2] FDPs are potent anticoagulants; they interfere with the action of thrombin, prevent normal polymerization of fibrin, and interfere with platelet function. All these responses promote generalized bleeding.

The normal coagulation process

In the normal vascular system, there is a balance between clot formation and clot dissolution.

Initial response

Following endothelial injury, hemostasis is achieved initially by vasoconstriction, which reduces the flow of blood. Simultaneously, platelets adhere to the damaged endothelial lining of the vessel and secrete both adenosine diphosphate (ADP) and catecholamines. Since ADP is a potent platelet adhesive factor, it attracts and

Table 9-1. Known Clotting Factors and Synonyms

FACTOR	SYNONYM
I	Fibrinogen
II	Prothrombin
III	Thromboplastin (tissue), extrinsic tissue activator
IV	Calcium
V	Accelerator globulin, proaccelerin, labile factor, cofactor of thromboplastin
VI	No longer used
VII	Proconvertin, serum prothrombin conversion accelerator (SPCA), stable factor, cothromboplastin
VIII	Antihemophiliac factor (AHF), platelet cofactor I, antihemophiliac globulin
IX	Christmas factor, antihemophiliac factor B, plasma thromboplastin component (PTC)
X	Stuart-Prower factor, Stuart factor
XI	Plasma thromboplastin antecedent (PTA)
XII	Hageman factor, contact factor
XIII	Fibrin-stabilizing factor, L-L factor, Laki-Lorand factor

Reprinted, with permission, from Leavell BS, Thorup OA: *Fundamentals of Clinical Hematology*, 4th ed, p 578. Philadelphia: Saunders, 1976.

binds additional free platelets, forming a platelet plug. Catecholamines induce the further release of ADP.

After this initial response, the coagulation system takes over. Fibrin, the final product of coagulation, consolidates with the platelet aggregate to strengthen the hemostatic plug at the bleeding site.

Clot formation

The coagulation system governs a complex sequence of reactions between proteins, lipids, and calcium ions (Figure 9-2). This sequence can be activated by two

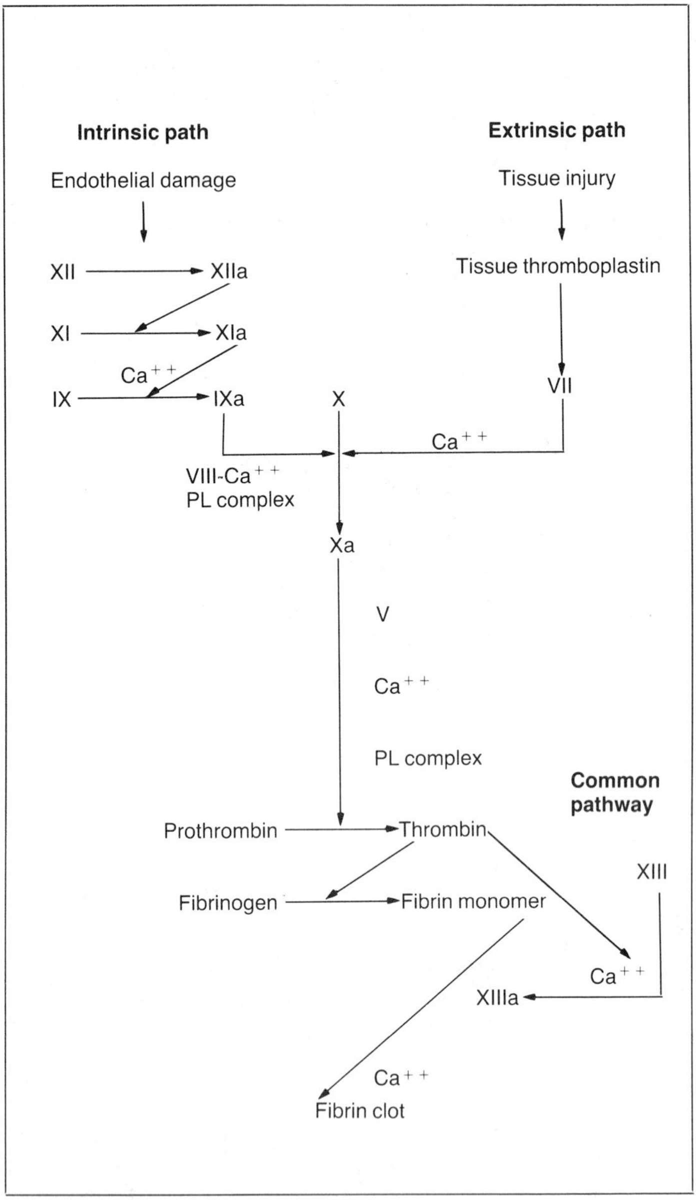

Figure 9-2. Formation of an insoluble fibrin clot. PL = phospholipid.

separate mechanisms. The first, or intrinsic, pathway begins with the activation of factor XII (Hageman factor) by contact of blood with exposed collagen or other foreign surfaces. The second, or extrinsic, pathway is initiated when thromboplastin, a lipoprotein released by injured tissue, joins with factor X in the blood. Factor X is the first step on the common pathway. After this step, prothrombin is converted to thrombin, and fibrinogen is converted to fibrin. Factor XIII (fibrin-stabilizing factor) finally catalyzes the cross-linking of fibrin monomers to produce a solid clot.[2]

Clot dissolution

Fibrinolysis, or clot dissolution, involves the conversion of the proenzyme plasminogen, a protein residing in the thrombus, to the active proteolytic enzyme plasmin. Plasmin acts on fibrinogen as well as on fibrin-producing fibrinogen degradation products.

Normally, the processes of clot formation and clot dissolution are in balance to prevent widespread coagulation or hemorrhage.

Other mechanisms

Other physiologic mechanisms play a role in controlling coagulation. Rapidly flowing blood reduces the concentration of activated coagulation factors by dilution. Excess coagulation factors—fibrin, fibrinogen degradation products, and endotoxins—are removed from the blood by the reticuloendothelial system.[4]

Causes and predisposing factors

DIC occurs as a complication of disorders such as shock, surgical procedures, respiratory distress syndrome, trauma, abruptio placentae or placenta previa, neoplasms, transfusion reactions, preeclampsia-eclampsia, retained fetal tissue, burns, vasculitis, dissecting aortic aneurysms, heat stroke, gram-negative septicemia, and viral infections. However, the exact cause of DIC is unknown. In all these disorders, there is disruption of vascular endothelium (which activates the intrinsic pathway) and tissue injury (resulting in the release of large amounts of thromboplastin into the circulation and activation of the extrinsic system). Damage to the vascular endothelium and tissue injury result in widespread intravascular clotting, fibrinolysis, and impairment of the reticuloendothelial system secondary to hypoperfusion.

Procoagulants

In severe tissue trauma (eg, crush injuries), tissue products may enter the circulation and trigger the coagulation mechanism; hypoxemia and hypotension may play a similar role. Other procoagulants, such as tumor cells, viruses, snake venom, bacterial endotoxins, and pancreatic enzymes, can also initiate a coagulopathy on entering the circulation.

Liver disease

Liver disease may lead to a deficiency of any or all of the clotting factors, creating disorders of hemostasis. A diseased or hypoperfused liver cannot remove activated clotting factors efficiently. This can result in an increase in fibrin degradation products, which interfere with platelet function.

Sepsis

Sepsis can trigger the coagulation process in a number of ways. This process may involve endothelial damage, damage to platelets caused by bacterial endotoxins, and activation of the coagulation system secondary to the interaction of endotoxin with leukocytes, releasing thromboplastin.

Other factors

Patients in shock have shown a decrease in coagulation factors from many causes: inadequate tissue perfusion, stagnant flow, endothelial damage, impaired kidney function, and decreased liver perfusion. Metabolic by-products also accumulate, with a resultant acidosis (a potent coagulation activator). Microthrombi can be found in the livers, kidneys, lungs, and hearts of patients dying of shock caused by hemorrhage, sepsis, or myocardial infarction. Despite this, hemorrhagic shock is not felt to produce clinically significant DIC, even in the presence of substantial hypotension and acidosis.[1] DIC may also follow cardiopulmonary bypass surgery.

Clinical features of DIC

Paradoxically, DIC involves both thrombosis and hemorrhage. The clinical signs may range from a transient drop in platelet count to life-threatening hemorrhage. Early clinical signs usually include bleeding from venipuncture or injection sites, mucous membranes, surgical incisions, drain sites, or tracheostomy sites or the appearance of petechiae, ecchymosis, or acrocyanosis. There may also be bleeding from the urinary tract or gastrointestinal tract. Diffuse bleeding in a patient with sepsis, shock, hypotension, crush injuries, or neoplasms strongly suggests DIC.

The organs most commonly involved in the clotting/bleeding process are the kidneys, skin, and lungs. Other organs that may be affected are the liver, pancreas, spleen, brain, heart, adrenal glands, and GI tract. The clinical signs and symptoms will depend upon the organ or system involved:

- Renal system: oliguria, anuria, hematuria
- Skin: acrocyanosis, purpura, ecchymosis
- Lungs: rales, dyspnea, cyanosis, hemoptysis

- Brain: disorientation, confusion, strokelike symptoms
- Heart: sudden onset of congestive heart failure
- GI tract: abdominal tenderness, sudden diarrhea, guaiac-positive stools, or emesis.

The severity of bleeding seems to be inversely related to the levels of fibrinogen and circulating platelets. The thrombotic manifestations may not be as obvious, for they occur primarily in the microcirculation.[1] Shock may be a sign of DIC as well as a predisposing cause.

Diagnosis

No test is specific to the diagnosis of DIC. The diagnosis is made on the basis of clinical assessment and the laboratory studies of coagulation (see Table 9-2).

The presence of fibrin degradation products will cause prolongation of the prothrombin time (PT) and partial thromboplastin time (PTT). Fibrin degradation products block the conversion of fibrinogen to fibrin, with resulting prolongation of the thrombin time. Thrombocytopenia develops because of the consumption of platelets in the forming of microthrombi.[1]

Treatment

The treatment of DIC depends on locating and treating the primary disease process. In addition, therapy to support life functions and to prevent or treat shock and acidosis should be instituted. The syndrome of DIC is especially difficult to treat because the contradictory problems of clotting and bleeding each require therapy that can exacerbate the other.[3] Other than treating the underlying disease process, few therapies are available.

Heparin may be used in the treatment of DIC. Heparin interrupts the cycle of thrombin release, fibrin deposition, clotting factor activation, and further thrombin release that characterizes DIC. Fibrinolysis will then cease and bleeding will subside. The risk of hemorrhage—from open wounds or other lesions—may sometimes outweigh the supposed benefits of heparin therapy.

There have been reports of thrombocytopenia and thrombotic complications related to the use of heparin.[5] At present, the tendency is to give heparin only if end-organ failure due to thrombosis is present or if the underlying disorder cannot be treated immediately.

The dose of heparin, if indicated, is controversial, since it is unclear what amount will be effective. The rec-

Table 9-2. Laboratory Studies of Coagulation

TEST	NORMAL	DIC
Platelet count	130,000 to 350,000	Decreased
Prothrombin time	12 to 15 seconds (control + 4 seconds)	Prolonged
Bleeding time	35 to 50 seconds	Prolonged
Partial thromboplastin time	(control + 10 seconds)	Prolonged
Fibrinogen	160 to 350 mg/100 mL	Decreased
Fibrinogen degradation products	0 to 10 μg/mL	Elevated
FM-FDP complex*		Positive
Thrombin time	12 seconds	Prolonged
Activated coagulation time	75 to 90 seconds	Prolonged
Factors II, VIII, V		Decreased
Ethanol gelation		Positive
Protamine sulfate		High titer
RBC fragments		Present

*Fibrin monomer-fibrin degradation product complex.

ommended dosage is 5,000 to 10,000 IU initially, followed by 1,000 to 1,500 IU hourly by continuous intravenous infusion.[4]

Therapy may be aimed at replacing the consumed clotting factors. Whole blood or blood components, platelets, fresh frozen plasma, and cryoprecipitates may be administered. This therapy carries the risk of adding fuel to the fire by stimulating more clotting. Heparin may be given first, to slow or stop the clotting process, before the clotting factors are replaced. The patient is also subjected to the small but serious risk of contracting hepatitis from blood and blood component therapy.

Nursing goals and interventions

The nursing management of a patient with DIC is complicated and challenging. The patient is critically ill, with multiple systems involved in the disease process(es). The bleeding may be subtle or overt. Evidence of thrombosis may be difficult to ascertain, since the symptoms will vary, depending on the organ involved and the degree of vascular obstruction. However, the earlier the problem is identified and treatment instituted, the better the prognosis.

In addition to care related to the underlying disease, the three main nursing goals for the patient with DIC are (1) early recognition of the bleeding/clotting disorder, (2) prevention of tissue trauma and unnecessary bleeding, and (3) prevention or early detection of further complications.

Early recognition of bleeding/clotting disorder

1. Identify patients at risk: patients with shock, sepsis, trauma, renal or liver dysfunction, or underlying blood disorders.

2. Assess patients at risk frequently:
   a. Hemodynamic parameters (drop in blood pressure, increase in heart rate, decrease in cardiac filling pressures, decrease in cardiac output)
   b. Laboratory values (decrease in Hct, Hb, and platelets; prolongation of PT, PTT, and TT; decrease in fibrinogen)
   c. Skin (petechiae or ecchymoses; bleeding at venipuncture, incision, or drainage sites)
   d. Respiratory system (presence of hemoptysis, rales, dyspnea; deterioration of blood gases)
   e. Cardiovascular system (signs and symptoms of congestive heart failure)
   f. Gastrointestinal system (guaiac-positive stools, nasogastric aspirate, or vomitus; abdominal pain; unexplained hypotension)
   g. Mucous membranes (epistaxis, bleeding gums)
   h. Central nervous system (change in level of consciousness, strokelike symptoms)
   i. Unusual drainage (oozing or frank bleeding from incisions or stab wounds, sump or Penrose drains, chest tubes, Foley catheter, or nasogastric tube).

Prevention of tissue trauma and unnecessary bleeding

1. Apply pressure to bleeding sites.
2. Do not disturb clots.
3. Avoid intramuscular injections. If needle sticks are necessary, use the smallest gauge needle and apply pressure. If possible, obtain blood samples from central venous lines or arterial lines.
4. Alert all staff members to the patient's condition when invasive procedures are being considered.
5. Prevent pressure areas; turn and position the patient frequently and gently to prevent trauma. Use a sheepskin, egg crate, or water mattress for cushioning.

6. Give frequent, gentle mouth care; prevent oral infections and use a soft toothbrush or gauze pads to prevent trauma.
7. Prevent respiratory complications by means of chest physiotherapy, adequate humidification, and sterile technique for suctioning.
8. Secure all drainage tubes to prevent unnecessary pulling and irritation.
9. Prevent infection by using aseptic technique in all dressing changes and invasive procedures.
10. Allay anxiety by explaining all procedures and routines. Be calm and reassuring.

Prevention or early detection of further complications

1. Be aware of drug reactions and interactions.
2. Monitor heparin and blood component therapy.
3. Monitor therapeutic effects of therapy.
4. Monitor for adverse effects of therapy.
5. Monitor laboratory values.
6. Prevent and/or treat acidosis.

Unfortunately, despite the best of nursing care, the mortality associated with DIC is high because the underlying disease often cannot be controlled. Therefore, nurses face another challenge: helping both patients and their families to cope with the stress of multiple, life-threatening illnesses.

REFERENCES

1. Rodman GH: Bleeding and clotting problems in the critically ill patient. In *Intensive Care Therapeutics* (Civetta JM, ed), p 150. New York: Appleton Century Crofts, 1980

2. Archibald LH, Keane B, Hafey L, Moody, FG: Complications of general surgery. In *Concepts and Practice of Intensive Care for Nurse Specialists* (Meltzer L, Abdellah FG, Kitchell JR, eds) 2nd ed, p 415. Bowie, Md: Charles Press, 1976

3. O'Brian BS, Woods S: The paradox of DIC. *Am J Nurs* 78:1878, 1978

4. Bart JB, Dear CB: Hematopoetic disorders. In *AACN's Clinical Reference for Critical Care Nursing*. p 594. New York: McGraw-Hill, 1981

5. Rice L, Jackson D: Can heparin cause clotting? *Heart Lung* 10:331, 1981

10

RENAL FAILURE

GEORGINA RANDOLPH, RN, MBA, MSN

The kidneys filter the blood, excrete the body's soluble waste, and control the volume and pressure of the body's fluids as well as their composition. The importance of the kidneys in maintaining homeostasis is comparable to that of the heart and brain; however, they are more vulnerable to the destructive effects of shock because their supply of blood is more rapidly compromised. This is evidenced by the oliguria so commonly seen in shock.

The body responds to the crisis of shock by instituting compensatory mechanisms that deflect the movement of blood from the nonvital areas, which are not in immediate need of blood to survive, to vital areas such as the brain and heart. Specifically, when pressoreceptors in the aorta and carotid artery sense a severe fall in blood pressure, they trigger the stimulation of the sympathetic nervous system. As a result, the adrenal glands release norepinephrine and epinephrine, causing vasoconstriction and a consequent reduction of blood flow to nonpriority areas such as the skin, gastrointestinal tract, liver, lungs, and kidneys.

The various body organs respond differently to this change in the distribution of blood. The first part of this chapter looks at the kidneys' ways of protecting themselves from the loss of perfusion. After that, nursing responsibilities are discussed, followed by a consideration of drug treatment and possible complications.

Renal autoregulation

Autoregulation is the intrinsic tendency of any organ to maintain a relatively constant flow of blood regardless of extrinsic factors such as variations in arterial pressure. In the kidneys specifically, blood flow remains proportional to mean arterial pressure as long as the latter stays between 90 and 240 mm Hg.

Autoregulation depends on changes in the resistance of the afferent and efferent arterioles, which respectively feed and drain the glomeruli. For example, in a patient whose hypovolemia is compensated, the afferent glomerular arteriole is dilated and the efferent arteriole constricted. Blood is filtered longer in the glomerulus (under lower pressure) and less water is passed in the filtrate, thus reducing the glomerular filtration rate (GFR). When less blood flows through the glomerular capillaries, the amount of filtrate in the proximal tubule decreases, and it flows more slowly through the tubule. Thus there is more time for sodium and water to be reabsorbed. The result is decreased urine volume and a higher specific gravity, both of which are seen in the patient's response to shock.

The renin-angiotensin system

Another regulatory mechanism is the renin-angiotensin system. When sympathetic vasoconstriction shunts blood away from the kidneys, the juxtaglomerular cells in the walls of the afferent arterioles release a substance called renin into the blood. Renin circulates in the blood, reacting with a substrate called angiotensinogen, a circulating polypeptide of hepatic origin, to produce angiotensin I. In the presence of a converting enzyme from lung tissue and probably from kidney tissue as well, angiotensin I is chemically altered to form angiotensin II.

Angiotensin II is a potent vasoconstrictor of both arteries and veins. This vasoconstriction increases blood pressure and facilitates venous return to the right side of the heart. Angiotensin II also stimulates the adenal cortex to release the mineralocorticoid aldosterone, which causes the kidneys to increase the reabsorption of sodium in the distal tubules. This, in turn, leads to the reabsorption of water under the influence of antidiuretic hormone (ADH). Thus the end results of the release of renin from the juxtaglomerular cells are (1) sodium and water retention, (2) decreased urine output, (3) increased fluid volume, and (4) increased blood pressure.

Intrarenal blood flow

Along with the greatly decreased flow of blood *to* the kidney in shock, there is also a great change in the blood flow *within* the kidney. Even in the early phases of circulatory collapse, blood is diverted from the renal cortex while flow to the medulla remains fairly constant. As shock progresses, the cortex becomes increasingly ischemic, but the medulla is perfused as long as possible. The purpose of this autoregulatory response is probably to preserve the function of the juxtamedullary nephrons. These are essential to the function of the countercurrent system, which concentrates the urine. If, with prolonged shock and continued cortical ischemia, the countercurrent mechanism fails, the urine becomes dilute and creatinine and osmolar clearances are markedly reduced. Soon after this dilute urine appears, there will be acute renal failure usually associated with acute tubular necrosis.

Renal responses to septic shock

Patients with shock due to sepsis may not have the typical renal responses already described. They may exhibit a syndrome of polyuria without azotemia, where the GFR may be slightly depressed but renal blood flow is increased and varies directly with cardiac output. Since this polyuria occurs with a low blood pressure and inadequate circulating volume, it is called "inappropriate diuresis." Apparently the normal renal compensatory mechanisms do not operate during early septic shock; instead, there is renal vasodilation. In this syndrome it is vitally important to replace the fluid that is lost; otherwise hypovolemia and acute renal failure are very likely to follow.

High-output renal insufficiency

In high-output renal insufficiency, another renal response to shock, the urine output is inappropriately high and there is azotemia. These patients will also have a low GFR, high serum creatinine, and low renal osmolar clearance, as do patients with renal insufficiency associated with oliguria. It has been postulated that high-output renal insufficiency is related to the successful early treatment of hypovolemic shock. Since the duration of insult to the kidneys is shortened, the response is diuresis rather than oliguria. Replacement therapy is, again, very critical, as is careful attention to fluid intake and output.

Oliguria

Oliguria exists when the urine flow is less than a stated minimum (eg, 400 mL/day for a 70-kg patient); it is the most common renal problem encountered in the patient with shock. A minimal output of 0.5 mL/kg/h will usually provide a sufficient margin of safety to permit excretion without azotemia during shock. However, urine flow of 0.8 to 1.0 mL/kg/h is more reliable.

Table 10-1. Clinical Findings Related to the Kidney in Shock

Early	↓ Urine output—reduced blood flow to nephrons
	↑ Urinary osmolarity—↑ ADH
	↓ Urinary sodium—aldosterone
	↑ Specific gravity—hormonal compensation
Late	↓ Urine output—below 0.5 mL/kg/h
	↓ Urine osmolarity—approaching the concentration of plasma
	↓ Specific gravity—kidneys lose their ability to concentrate and excrete waste products

When oliguria develops despite adequate hydration, immediate measures to prevent renal shutdown are required. However, no diuretic or osmotic agent can prevent kidney failure if the underlying cause is not treated.

Nursing responsibilities

With regard to shock, your first responsibility is to recognize the clinical manifestations of the body's compensatory mechanisms. Clinical findings related to the kidney are outlined in Table 10-1. Your second major task is to identify patients at risk for shock and monitor urine function closely. These responsibilities are discussed below.

Assessment

Nursing assessment—based on both clinical findings and laboratory data—is an ongoing process that provides a basis for comparison and gives a continual picture of the patient's compensatory status. Frequent assessment is critical to establish baselines and document trends—both of which are far more valuable than single measurements.

Input/output records

In the care of patients with kidney problems, careful attention to fluid balance (ie, accurate and complete intake/output records) is of major importance. Urine output can also be used to evaluate fluid replacement.

Renal function is assessed by measuring and recording hourly urine output and specific gravity. An indwelling Foley catheter connected to a urometer ensures the accurate measurement of urine. Urine output is an accurate indicator of renal perfusion, since output decreases if perfusion pressure is not adequate for filtration.

Hidden fluid losses. Consideration must also be given to unmeasured or hidden fluid losses, such as insensible fluid loss, profuse perspiration, and copious drainage from any site. Fractures, for example, can cause blood loss into the surrounding soft tissue without gross evidence. Massive internal fluid loss into body spaces (eg, retropleural bleeding, hemothorax, peritoneal bleeding, bleeding into the gastrointestinal lumen) can also occur. Considerable fluid can also drain onto dressings; they, too, must be evaluated. This can be done by weighing wet dressings.

Weight measurement. To ensure the accuracy of daily weight measurements, they should be obtained on the same scale at the same time of day with the patient wearing the same amount of clothing.

Blood pressure. Blood pressure should be monitored and maintained at a level sufficient to produce a urine flow of at least 0.5 mL/kg/h—the minimal amount sufficient to avoid azotemia, as already mentioned.

Other indicators

Other indicators of renal function, determined by laboratory tests, are outlined in Table 10-2.

Treatment goals

The main goal of treatment in renal failure is to maintain an optimal level of hydration with an adequate circulating blood volume so as to reinstate renal blood flow and prevent necrotic damage.

Plan

To support renal blood flow, use
- Fluids to expand volume
- Diuretics to draw interstitial fluid into the bloodstream
- Catecholamines to increase renal blood flow.

Again, it is important to monitor the patient continuously and to watch for possible fluid overload.

Table 10-2. Laboratory Tests to Assess Kidney Function

TEST	NORMAL VALUES	CHANGES IN SHOCK
Urine		
Creatinine clearance	♂ 1.0-2.0 g/24 h ♀ 0.8-1.8 g/24 h	↓—impaired renal excretion
Osmolarity	500-800 mosm/mL	↑ Early—water retention secondary to ADH ↓ Late—inability of kidneys to concentrate urine
Specific gravity	1.001-1.035	↑ Early—as above ↓ Late—influenced by administration of dextran
Sodium	80-100 mEq/24 h	↓ Early—sodium reabsorption secondary to aldosterone ↓ or ↑ late—abnormal renal function
Potassium	40-80 mEq/24 h	↑ Early—due to K^+ excretion secondary to aldosterone ↓ or ↑ late—due to abnormal renal function GI bleeding Infection
Blood		
BUN	10-12 mg/dL	↑ Protein intake Renal failure
Creatinine	0.1-2.0 mg/dL	↑ In renal failure

Outcome criteria

- Urinary output of 30 to 60 mL/h
- Urine specific gravity of 1.010 to 1.025
- Stable weight.

Fluid replacement

Patients in shock must have adequate fluid volume if other treatments are to be effective in restoring tissue perfusion. The appropriate replacement fluid remains controversial. Blood is the only fluid that can restore oxygen-carrying capacity. It also contains protein, which contributes to the maintenance of osmotic pressure. However, replacement with whole blood presents difficulties and dangers. Chapter 4, on hypovolemic shock, discusses the specifics of fluid and electrolyte replacement in detail.

Drugs and renal response

Hypovolemia must be treated before any sympathomimetic drug is administered. Urine output is a good indicator of the effectiveness of therapy. Assess output hourly and look for a minimum of 30 mL/h.

Dopamine

In low doses (usually 3 to 7 μg/kg/min), dopamine (Intropin) increases renal perfusion by stimulating vasodilation and thus increasing renal blood flow. Prognosis is more favorable when therapy is begun early, especially before urine flow drops below 20 mL/h.

Dobutamine

Dobutamine (Dobutrex) is the drug of choice for cardiac decompensation. It does not cause renal dilation, as does dopamine. Since it increases cardiac output, it may also increase the flow of blood to the kidneys.

Mannitol and furosemide

Mannitol (12.5–25 g IV) exerts an osmotic pull to draw fluid into the intravascular space, and it may also help to protect cell membranes. It produces an obligatory urine flow by interfering with the nephron transport mechanism. Mannitol is freely filtered but not reabsorbed by the kidneys; thus its excretion carries with it increased amounts of water. If mannitol fails, furosemide (Lasix) 5–10 mg IV may be tried. This powerful loop diuretic is also an electrolyte depleter, so close monitoring of serum Na^+ and K^+ is necessary. Furosemide inhibits the active reabsorption of sodium in the proximal tubule and should therefore be used only *after* blood volume has been restored.

Possible complications of renal ischemia

With prolonged vasoconstriction, oxygen delivery to the nephrons, especially those in the outer cortical areas, becomes inadequate. As a result, the nephrons' tubular cells suffer damage and the nephrons themselves cannot continue their work of filtration, secretion, and reabsorption. The tubular cells may die, slough off into the lumen, and thus further impair tubular flow. Acute tubular necrosis ensues, leading to acute renal failure.

When the diagnosis of acute renal failure has been established, dialysis is begun at once in order to prevent uremia. The procedure is repeated at frequent intervals—even daily—until renal function returns. Frequent dialysis also facilitates nutritional therapy. Unless they have had abdominal surgery, hemodynamically unstable patients usually tolerate peritoneal dialysis well.

Summary

The kidneys are especially vulnerable to shock, yet preservation of renal function is important to recovery. This chapter has stressed the importance of oliguria as a sign of renal impairment. However, it is important to realize that a normal or high urine flow is no guarantee of normal kidney function. Other parameters (such as the BUN and creatinine concentrations) must be evaluated in addition if renal status is to be properly monitored and maintained.

BIBLIOGRAPHY

Hurley EJ: Hypovolemic shock. In *Current Practice in Critical Care.* St Louis: Mosby, 1979

Petlin A, Carolan J: Halt hypovolemic shock. *RN,* May 1982, p 36

Rice V: Shock, a clinical syndrome. *Crit Care Nurs,* 1981

Wilson R: Shock, its definition, classification, diagnosis, pathophysiology, monitoring and treatment. In *A Manual of Practice and Techniques* in *Critical Care Medicine,* 1976

Zschoche DA, ed: *Mosby's Comprehensive Review of Critical Care,* 2nd ed. St Louis: Mosby, 1980

11

TEMPERATURE RESPONSES IN SHOCK

RHONDA M. WELLER, RN, MSN

All the various types of shock discussed in the earlier chapters of this book have the same end result: inadequate perfusion of vital body tissues. In response, the body calls on a number of compensatory mechanisms which, among other things, destabilize the body's temperature. That is, the normal balance between the heat produced by body metabolism and that lost to the surroundings is disturbed. The pattern of this disturbance depends on the type and stage of shock.

Hypovolemic and cardiogenic shock

Although the precipitating causes of these two types of shock differ (inadequate volume versus inadequate pumping ability), both hypovolemic and cardiogenic shock (see Chapters 4 and 6) result in decreased stroke volume, cardiac output, and blood pressure. The fall in blood pressure stimulates pressoreceptors in the aorta and the carotid arteries, which signal the vasomotor center in the medulla oblongata. This center, in turn, stimulates the sympathetic branch of the autonomic nervous system, causing widespread constriction of the vessels supplying the skin, gastrointestinal tract, and kidneys and shunting of blood preferentially to the body's most vital organs, the heart and brain. It is this phenomenon that affects body temperature.

Decreased blood flow to the skin means that less heat is conducted from the body's core to its surface. Hence the patient's skin will characteristically be both pale and cold. The low skin temperature will lead to a decrease in body temperature unless heat production is increased. Therefore, sensors at the periphery signal the hypothalamic thermostat to alter its "set point," which is then driven to the threshold of shivering even though the temperature of the hypothalamus itself is within normal limits. By shivering, the body attempts to increase heat production in anticipation of a drop in internal temperature. As a result, the core body temperature of the patient in shock will initially be close to normal.

Moist skin in patients with hypovolemic or cardiogenic shock does not represent an attempt by the body to rid itself of excess heat. Instead, this moisture results from the effect of increased circulating levels of epinephrine and norepinephrine, which can cause sympathetic stimulation of the sweat glands.

In trying to keep its temperature within normal limits, the body sets to work mechanisms—notably shivering—that increase its metabolic rate. This calls for increased use of oxygen at a time when the oxygen supply to the tissues is already compromised. At the same time, cellular metabolic demands are being increased by the effects of increased circulating catecholamines. If tissue perfusion is further reduced by prolonged vasoconstriction, the cellular deficit of oxygen will decrease the production of adenosine triphosphate (ATP) and increase anaerobic metabolism. The result will be metabolic acidosis, which will further undermine cellular functioning.

This apparently complex sequence of events has a very simple result: Less body heat is generated. Core body temperature then drops and recorded temperature is usually subnormal. If, during this progressive phase of shock, peripheral vasoconstriction can be reduced and cardiac output increased, body temperature may return to normal.

If, however, cardiac output and blood pressure fall below critical levels, cerebral blood flow will be impaired, resulting in cerebral ischemia.[1] This decrease in cerebral perfusion causes a sympathetic vasomotor discharge that is seven times stronger than the discharge elicited by the pressoreceptors.[2] In the final stages of refractory, or irreversible, shock, cerebral ischemia depresses the brain's vital centers. At this point, the temperature-regulatory function of the hypothalamus becomes totally ineffective, further heat loss often ensues, and the patient falls into a coma. Shivering now ceases.

Neurogenic shock

If injury to the spine occurs above the area of sympathetic outflow from the cord, regulation of body temperature is seriously affected by poikilothermia, a state in which the hypothalamus loses its ability to control both perfusion to the skin and sweating. Therefore the patient's temperature will approach that of the surrounding environment. For this reason, it is vital to protect all patients in shock from extremes of environmental temperature.)

Anaphylactic shock

Anaphylactic shock (see Chapter 8) is due to an antigen-antibody reaction that causes damage to tissues and release of histamine, a potent vasodilator. Generally, a pattern of low-grade temperature elevation is seen, since injected pyrogens do not immediately reset the hypothalamic thermostat. They must react with polymorphonuclear leukocytes, monocytes, and certain reticuloendothelial cells to form endogenous pyrogen before they affect the body temperature. In any event, fever is a relatively minor problem in this form of shock, which can have many more serious, life-threatening consequences.

Septic shock

Septic shock (see Chapter 5) is caused by the depressive effect of toxins released by bacteria. In this form of shock, the temperature may rise as high as 105° or 106°F or it may fall below normal, depending on the stage of shock and the causative organism. In gram-negative sepsis, the most common kind, two very different clinical pictures emerge. These are "warm," or high-output, shock and "cold," or low-output, shock.

Warm shock

Typically, body temperature is likely to be elevated in warm shock. This is due to the toxins' ability to act as pyrogens, causing the set point of the hypothalamic thermostat to rise. This brings all the mechanisms for raising body temperature into play, including the conservation of heat and production of additional body heat to raise the body temperature to the new, higher level.

While the blood is being warmed to the new high, however, the patient experiences chills and feels cold. The skin is cold because of vasoconstriction; the patient shivers in an attempt to produce additional heat. Until the body temperature reaches the new set point, the chills will continue. When the new value is finally attained, the patient feels neither cold nor hot.

If the factor causing the elevation in temperature is removed, the hypothalamic thermostat is reset at a lower level, causing the body to try to rid itself of heat through vasodilation and intense sweating. This reversal of the febrile response is frequently referred to as the crisis, or "flush."[1]

Cold shock

If the shock persists, the second type of septic shock develops, in which venous return to the heart, stroke volume and cardiac output, and tissue perfusion are all decreased. As in the case of hypovolemic or cardiogenic shock, the blood pressure falls and tissue perfusion is compromised; the result is a decrease in surface temperature. Commonly, as continued metabolic derangements lead to irreversible shock, the body temperature once again declines to subnormal levels.

Nursing care

The nurse plays an important role in the prevention of shock. Careful observation of patients known to be at risk may lead to the institution of appropriate therapies in time to avert more serious complications.

In the critically ill patient, temperature should be monitored at least every 4 hours, more frequently if necessary. Rectal measurements are generally considered to be the safest as well as the most accurate measure of core temperature. Surface temperature may vary with the temperature of the surrounding environment. Both surface skin temperature and skin color should be monitored continually; pale, cold skin indicates intense vasoconstriction. Recently, peripheral skin perfusion has been assessed quite accurately by measuring the toe temperature of patients in shock. In one study,[3] toe temperature was shown to be a better indicator of survival in cardiogenic shock than blood lactate, cardiac index, or arterial pressure. Measurement of toe temperature is felt to provide an inexpensive, simple, noninvasive, and quantitative indicator of the severity of cardiogenic shock.

The most serious consequence of fever is derangement of the enzymatic reactions necessary to sustain life. In addition, there is a sevenfold increase in the tissues' oxygen requirements for every degree (Fahrenheit) of increased temperature. This phenomenon renders the brain vulnerable to hypoxia, which may sometimes be forestalled through the use of external cooling and the administration of oxygen.

Although a slight fever after surgery is not unusual and commonly lasts for several days, fever is often a sign of developing complications and should be brought to the attention of the physician. In order to control fever, tepid alcohol sponge baths, antipyretics, or ice bags may be used, in addition to hypothermia to produce cooling. Cooling with a hypothermia unit should be accomplished slowly in order to prevent a precipitous drop in temperature. Body temperature should be monitored at least every 30 minutes while cooling; other vital signs should be watched closely as well. Usually, temperature will continue to fall an additional degree or two after cooling is stopped. The patient should not be cooled to the point of shivering, which actually increases heat production.

Shivering, if it occurs, can be controlled with chlorpromazine (Thorazine) or diazepam (Valium) if the physician orders it. Give meticulous skin care and take comfort measures—eg, applying mineral oil, wrapping the knees and elbows with Kerlix dressings, and turning every 2 hours—to prevent complications associated with hypothermia. To facilitate cooling, keep only a bath blanket between the patient and the hypothermia unit.

Hypothermia may also be used to reduce metabolic rate during surgery. Shock, general anesthesia, and accidental environmental exposure lower the metabolic rate, slow the circulation, and may cause hypothermia. Administering cold fluids during resuscitation may also induce hypothermia. When the patient is to be warmed, it should be done slowly, with care to prevent skin trauma as well as overheating.

Knowledge of the patient and the surrounding circumstances is invaluable in determining appropriate therapeutic measures. For example, warming of a vasoconstricted patient can produce disastrous results. As vasodilation occurs, a profound drop in stroke volume, cardiac output, and blood pressure may result, further aggravating the state of shock.

Fever is usually, but not always, present in the septic patient. Sudden fever over 101°F accompanied by chills, lethargy, confusion, hyperventilation, tachycardia, and a drop in systolic blood pressure to less than 80 signals the onset of septic shock. On the other hand, the patient who is immunosuppressed, very young, or very old may never become febrile. Patients who are subjected to numerous venipunctures or the use of multiple invasive procedures challenge the nurse to deliver the utmost by way of aseptic preventive care. The patient with a spinal cord injury may have lost the ability to regulate temperature, necessitating the use of special protective measures. In nearly every patient, the potential for the development of a shock syndrome exists. It is therefore imperative that you possess well-developed powers of observation and assessment in order to provide the best possible care in both the prevention and treatment of shock.

REFERENCES

1. Guyton AC: *Textbook of Medical Physiology,* 6th ed. Philadelphia: Saunders, 1981

2. Berne RM, Levy MN: *Physiology.* St Louis: Mosby, 1983

3. Henning RJ, Wiener F, Valdes S, et al: Measurement of toe temperature for assessing the severity of acute circulatory failure. *Surg Gynecol Obstet* 149:1, 1979

GENERAL REFERENCES

Bordicks K: *Patterns of Shock: Implications for Nursing Care.* New York: Macmillan, 1965

Burrell LO, Burrell ZL: *Critical Care,* 4th ed. St Louis: Mosby, 1982

Chaney P (ed): *Assessing Vital Signs Accurately.* Horsham, Pa: Intermed Communications, 1977

Condon R, De Casse J: *Surgical Care, a Physiologic Approach to Clinical Management.* Philadelphia: Lea & Febiger, 1980

Haymaker W, Anderson E, Nauta W: *The Hypothalamus.* Springfield, Ill: Thomas, 1969

Kluger M: Temperature regulation, fever, and disease. In *International Review of Physiology, Environmental Physiology III* (Robertshaw D, ed). Baltimore: University Park Press, 1979

Rice V: Shock: A clinical syndrome, Part I. *Critical Care Nurse,* p 44, March-April 1981

Rice V: Shock: A clinical syndrome, Part II. *Critical Care Nurse,* p 4, May-June 1981

Rice V: Shock: A clinical syndrome, Part III. *Critical Care Nurse,* p 36, July-August 1981

Rice V: Shock: A clinical syndrome, Part IV. *Critical Care Nurse,* p 34, September-October 1981

Robinson J (ed): *Coping With Neurological Problems Proficiently.* Horsham, Pa: Intermed Communications, 1979

Schumer W, Kukral J: Metabolism of shock. *Surgery* 63:630, 1968

Seal A: *Cardiogenic Shock.* New York: Appleton-Century-Crofts, 1980

Shires G, Carrico C, Canizaro P: Shock. In *Major Problems in Clinical Surgery* (Dunphy J, ed). Philadelphia: Saunders, 1973

Underhill S, Wood S, Swarajan E, Halpenny C: *Cardiac Nursing.* Philadelphia: Lippincott, 1982

Wilson R: The diagnosis and management of severe sepsis and septic shock. *Heart Lung* 5:422, 1976

Zweifach B, Fronek A: The interplay of central and peripheral factors in irreversible hemorrhagic shock. *Progr Cardiovasc Dis* 17:147, 1975

12

ADRENAL RESPONSES IN SHOCK

KATHLEEN SCANLON, RN

Whenever homeostasis is threatened, as in shock, the body responds with a "fight or flight" reaction, in which the endocrine system plays an important role. Both the nervous and endocrine systems comprise an essential communications network that responds to crisis long before any clinical signs of shock become evident.

Physiologic response

Under stress, the body's first priority is to maintain adequate perfusion to the vital organs. Therefore, to protect cardiovascular integrity, it activates the negative feedback system represented in Figure 12-1.

Negative feedback system

As the diagram in Figure 12-1 shows, the first step in the sequence occurs when the sympathetic nervous system perceives the decreased cardiac output and immediately signals the anterior pituitary to secrete adrenocorticotropic hormone (ACTH). This hormone then stimulates the adrenal cortex to secrete the glucocorticoid cortisol. In addition to its antiinflammatory effects and stabilizing influence on carbohydrate metabolism, cortisol exerts a positive inotropic effect on the heart, enhancing cardiac output.

The decrease in cardiac output also stimulates a sympathoadrenal response whereby the catecholamines epinephrine and norepinephrine are released from the adrenal medulla (Figure 12-1, left). These hormones work to increase the effectiveness of the heart. Epinephrine has both inotropic and chronotropic effects on cardiac function, stimulating the beta receptors of the sympathetic nervous system and thereby increasing the rate and force of the heartbeat.

Norepinephrine causes vasoconstriction in the skeletal muscles, skin, and viscera when the alpha receptors

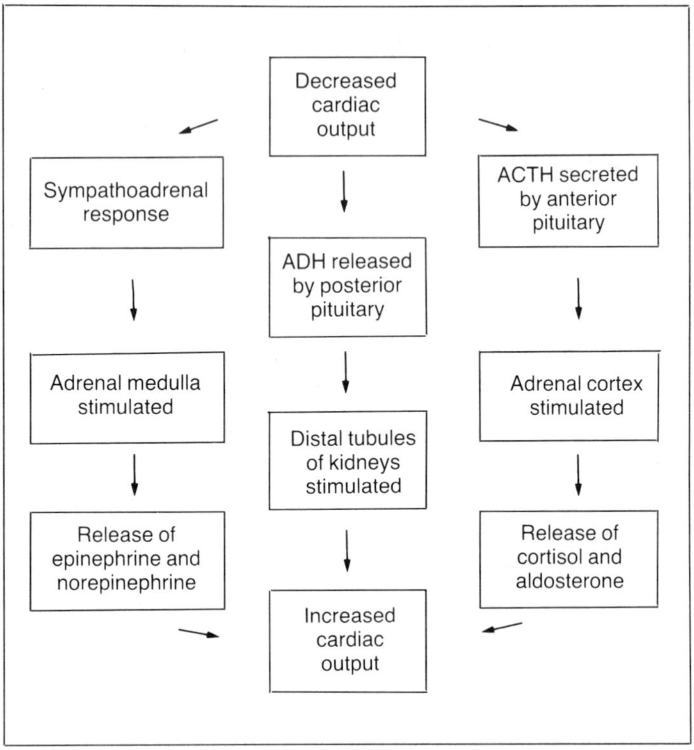

Figure 12-1. The negative feedback system protecting cardiovascular integrity.

in these areas are stimulated. As a result, there is a marked increase in peripheral resistance and the arterial blood pressure rises.

Antidiuretic hormone (ADH) is released from the posterior pituitary as serum osmolality declines. This hormone acts upon the distal tubules of the kidneys, promoting reabsorption of water so as to increase the fluid volume within the vasculature.

As renal perfusion declines, the adrenal cortex secretes aldosterone. As a result, sodium and water are retained in yet another effort to increase blood volume (Table 12-1).

Table 12-1. Primary Hormonal Intervention in Shock

HORMONE	SOURCE	MAJOR EFFECTS
ACTH	Anterior pituitary	Stimulates adrenal cortex to release epinephrine and norepinephrine
ADH	Posterior pituitary	Acts on distal tubules of kidneys, promoting reabsorption of water to increase fluid volume within the vasculature
Aldosterone	Adrenal cortex	Promotes retention of sodium and water in an effort to increase blood volume
Cortisol	Adrenal cortex	Acts as a positive inotropic agent to increase cardiac output. Antiinflammatory effect
Epinephrine	Adrenal medulla	Has positive inotropic and chronotropic effects, increasing rate and force of cardiac contractions
Norepinephrine	Adrenal medulla	Has a vasoconstrictive effect on skeletal muscles, skin, and viscera, increasing peripheral resistance and, with it, arterial blood pressure

Other humoral substances controlled by the sympathoadrenal system and cardiovascular mechanoreceptors include kinins, serotonin, histamine, prostacyclin, and thromboxane A_2; these hormones have direct cardiovascular and renal effects. Indirectly, they alter central or peripheral adrenergic transmission and promote the release of the neurotransmitter norepinephrine at the adrenergic terminal.

This negative feedback system is indispensable to preserving homeostasis; its effectiveness, however, is limited.

Regardless of the severity of the insult, the negative feedback system is activated in the same way and strives to maintain adequate blood flow to the vital organs by causing vasoconstriction within the vasculature of less vital areas. This response may be adequate when the injury is not severe or prolonged. An extensive insult, however, causes the system to remain activated indefinitely, producing a dangerous chain of events.

Positive feedback system

Extreme vasoconstriction results in poorly perfused tissues. Since the cells are not being adequately oxygenat-

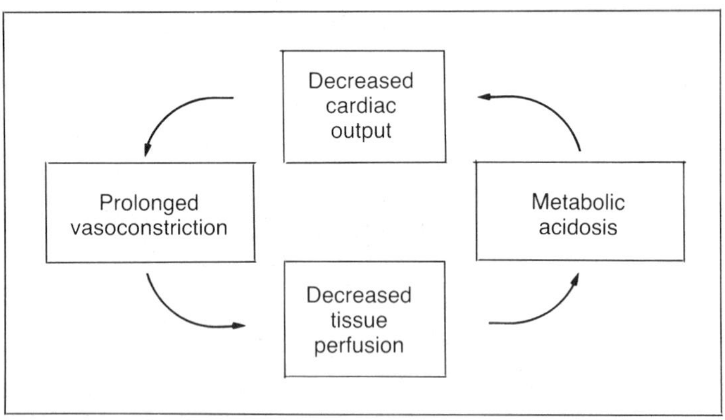

Figure 12-2. Positive feedback system characteristic of late-stage shock.

ed, they must resort to anaerobic metabolism, which leads to metabolic acidosis. At this point the negative feedback system turns positive (Figure 12-2), having become unable to maintain perfusion because of a sustained volume deficit, pump failure, or disruption of the neurohormonal response. A vicious cycle now ensues whereby the diminished flow of blood perpetuates vasoconstriction, thereby fostering the acidotic state and leading directly to death.

Nursing implications

Two critical implications in caring for a patient in shock are those of anticipation and time. These are especially relevant with regard to the endocrine system in shock, where timely intervention can prove to be lifesaving.

Assessment phase

The initial assessment should serve to establish the patient's current status while also providing a baseline for future reference.

Although it is useful to be able to recognize the clinical signs of shock, it is even more important to perceive the *potential* for shock. This is accomplished by way of a thorough physical assessment and history and the subsequent correlation of these with the known aspects of endocrine function.

Planning phase

In formulating a plan of care, it is important to remember that by the time deterioration becomes evident, the body has already reached a dangerous phase in its compensatory efforts. One implication of this fact is that caution is in order even in planning care for an apparently stable patient. In other words, the best plan of care will be flexible enough to allow for every contingency.

Standardize your initial plan for any patient by providing for the maintenance of airway, breathing, and circulation—the ABCs of resuscitation. Noting their presence and quality during the assessment phase and planning for routine observation is not enough. You must also focus your attention on how to support these vital areas should the need occur. Ask and answer hypothetical questions such as these: What actions should I take in the event of respiratory distress? Severe hypotension? Cardiac arrhythmias?

The planning phase is the time for organization and anticipation. It is essential to set priorities according to the data collected in the assessment phase and to create a workable plan for intervention. However, attention also needs to be paid to potential emergencies. It is much easier to plan for the worst possible eventuality than to be caught unaware.

Intervention phase

When signs of shock appear, it is obvious that the body has put its emergency response systems into effect. Since they can function only for a limited time, however, immediate medical intervention becomes imperative.

The primary nursing goals should be to support oxygenation and maintain adequate circulation. Intervention at this time demands:

1. Provision of an adequate airway
2. Sufficient oxygenation
3. Adequate circulatory volume
4. Maintenance of circulation
5. Correction of respiratory or metabolic acid-base and electrolyte imbalances.

Maintaining an adequate airway and supporting oxygenation may range from applying external oxygen delivery equipment to preparing for endotracheal intubation and ventilatory assistance.

Aside from noting the type and quality of respirations and the presence or absence of cyanosis, arterial blood gas readings are necessary to determine the degree of oxygenation and, just as important, ventilation. It may be possible to raise the PaO_2 with oxygen therapy, but if the patient's $PaCO_2$ is dangerously elevated, indicating impairment of gas exchange, ventilatory assistance may be necessary. Of course, severe respiratory distress will probably require immediate intubation with subsequent arterial blood gas measurements to evaluate treatment.

An adequate circulating volume is generally maintained by administering crystalloids (IV solution) and colloids (blood and/or albumin). It is always preferable to administer large quantities of fluid via a central line. In an emergency, large-bore peripheral lines will do, but make certain to watch for infiltration at the sites.

When administering fluids rapidly, check periodically for indications that the therapy is working and for indications of circulatory overload. A rise in blood pressure and central venous pressure (if available) mean that fluid resuscitation is successful. Ideally, pulmonary artery pressures give the best indications of the body's response to fluid therapy but often are not available at the onset of an emergency.

Vasopressor therapy is indicated when a circulatory volume is adequate but perfusion is not. Dopamine (Intropin) is used frequently to increase myocardial contractility, which in turn augments cardiac output. Low-dose dopamine, 2 to 5 μg/kg, has a direct effect on renal perfusion with little effect on blood pressure. Dosages of 5 to 10 μg/kg are more effective in raising blood pressure and still provide adequate peripheral perfusion. In severe cases, doses as high as 20 to 25 μg/kg may be needed to maintain a systolic blood pressure of 90 to 100 mm Hg. At this dosage range, vasoconstriction occurs, resulting in decreased renal perfusion as evidenced by a drop in urine output.

As discussed earlier, any type of uninterrupted shock eventually results in severe metabolic acidosis, which, if not corrected, ends in death. For this reason, corticosteroids are often administered in an attempt to support the microcirculation and therefore reverse the acidotic state.

Methylprednisolone (Solu-Medrol) is often given in a large dose initially of 1 g IV and then 100 to 250 mg IV at 2- to 6-hour intervals. Large IV doses should be given over 3 to 15 minutes to prevent cardiac arrhythmias and circulatory collapse.

Hydrocortisone (Solu-Cortef) is indicated immediately for adrenally insufficient patients who have gone into acute adrenal crisis. This can be due to abrupt cessation of corticosteroids in patients on long-term supplements or to stressors such as infection, trauma, or surgery. Initially 100 to 200 mg of hydrocortisone will be ordered IV push with subsequent administration via IV fluids, 100 mg/1,000 mL, to equal 800 mg within the first 24 hours (soluble hydrocortisone has a short half-life, so must be administered in an elevated dosage). Dosages will be decreased daily, depending on the patient's response to therapy.

Finally, correction of acid-base and electrolyte imbalances is imperative to the resolution of shock. Arterial and venous blood sampling will be required to obtain initial baseline values and subsequently to monitor the effectiveness of treatment.

Sodium bicarbonate is indicated to maintain a pH greater than 7.25 and a bicarbonate level of 20 to 25 mEq/L. Usually one ampoule (44 mEq) is given IV push every 10 minutes.

Both hyperkalemia and hypokalemia (normal serum potassium range is 3.5 to 5.3 mEq/L) may lead to dangerous cardiac arrhythmias. Hyperkalemia is generally seen early in shock but may soon be corrected by various resuscitative measures: rehydration with IV saline, administration of sodium bicarbonate (promotes transfer of potassium from extracellular to intracellular sites), or high-dose hydrocortisone therapy (promotes potassium excretion).

Initially hyperkalemia may swiftly change to hypokalemia, a development that requires IV potassium supplements. Frequently a potassium challenge (20 to 40 mEq in 100 to 250 mL over 1 to 3 h IV) will be given in an attempt to normalize the serum level, followed by maintenance doses (20 to 40 mEq/L). Potassium should always be administered slowly as a dilute solution, no more than 80 mEq/L and no faster than 20 mEq/h.

Successful intervention demands that you be one step ahead of developments at all times. This is accomplished by careful assessment and planning along with flexibility and foresight.

Evaluation phase

Whatever the outcome of a specific intervention may be, it is always useful to review it calmly, after the fact, since experience assimilated with intelligence is the best teacher. In other words, when theoretical knowledge and clinical skills are tested in practice and later reviewed, the expertise that can save lives will develop.

GENERAL REFERENCES

Beeson PB, McDermott W, Wyngaarden JB: *Cecil Textbook of Medicine,* 15th ed, p 1111. Philadelphia: Saunders, 1979

Beyers M, Dudas S: *The Clinical Practice of Medical-Surgical Nursing,* p 1183. Boston: Little, Brown, 1977

Brunner LS, Suddarth DS: *The Lippincott Manual of Nursing Practice,* 3rd ed. Philadelphia: Lippincott, 1982

Burrell LO, Burrell ZL: *Critical Care,* 4th ed, p 453. St Louis: Mosby, 1982

Chaffee E, Giersheimer E: *Basic Physiology and Anatomy,* 2nd ed, p 546. Philadelphia: Lippincott, 1969

Guyton AC: *Textbook of Medical Physiology,* 6th ed, ch 28. Philadelphia: Saunders, 1981

Kenner CV, Guzzetta CE, Dossey BM: *Critical Care Nursing: Body—Mind—Spirit,* pp 578, 768. Boston: Little, Brown, 1981

Niedringhaus L: A nursing emergency . . . Acute adrenal crisis. *Focus on Critical Care* 10(1): 30, February 1983

Nurse's guide to drugs. *Nursing '80,* pp 410, 570, 689, 694, 1980

Widmann FK: *Clinical Interpretation of Laboratory Tests,* pp 276, 278. Philadelphia: Davis, 1983

13

NUTRITION IN SHOCK

JACQUELINE M. CAROLAN, RN, BSN, CCRN

In-hospital malnutrition

An often-overlooked problem of patients in shock is malnutrition. Among adult patients in this category, nutritional needs to maintain energy may be increased by 10 to 100%, depending on the severity of trauma or disease. Elective surgery can increase energy demands by as much as 10%, multiple fractures by 10 to 30%, peritonitis by 30 to 50%, and severe burns by 30 to 100%.

Patients in shock may suffer progressive loss of both lean body mass and adipose tissue from inadequate intake of proteins and calories. Many who are admitted in acute shock have some nutritional reserve; patients who have little or none develop clinical signs of starvation more rapidly. Left untreated, malnutrition tends to increase morbidity and mortality.

Sources of energy

Fats, carbohydrates, and proteins are our three main sources of energy.

Fats. Fat, stored as triglycerides in adipose tissue, represents the body's largest amount of reserve energy. However, it cannot adequately satisfy the energy requirements of glucose-dependent metabolism, especially the brain, leukocytes, and granulation tissue.

Carbohydrates. The energy for glucose-dependent organs is supplied chiefly by carbohydrates, stored as glycogen in the liver and muscles. The calories from these sources, however, are exhausted within 16 to 24 hours after the onset of starvation.

Proteins. Proteins, unlike fats and carbohydrates, cannot be used for energy without diminishing the ability to respond to stress. Protein is stored in somatic and visceral forms. If the somatic stores are lost, the functions of both skeletal and smooth muscle are altered. If the visceral stores are depleted, changes are seen in plasma proteins as well as in antibodies and enzymes.

Losses during starvation

Early in starvation, a striking catabolic response occurs in the otherwise healthy patient. There is a marked increase in urinary losses of nitrogen, creatinine, and electrolytes and a caloric expenditure at times exceeding 6,000 kcal/day. Both protein anabolism and catabolism are accelerated, but catabolism is accelerated to a much greater degree. Protein loss represents increases both in the breakdown of body protein and in the synthesis of urea. Usually, a decrease in protein and calorie intake accompanies this catabolism.

During the first week of total starvation, the average person loses 4 to 5 kg of body weight; about 25% of this loss represents adipose tissue.

Assessment of patient status

The best treatment is, of course, prevention. On admission, therefore, all patients should be assessed nutritionally so that therapy can be tailored to their needs. In this assessment, both somatic and visceral proteins are measured. Somatic protein measurements reflect muscle status, whereas visceral protein measurements indicate the status of nonmuscle protein levels.

Height and weight

The first step in measuring somatic protein is to get the patient's height and weight. If a patient's weight is below 90% of the ideal for his height, nutritional support should be instituted. Patients must be weighed daily in order to evaluate trends.

When a patient's albumin is below 2.8 g/dL, it should be suspected that some of his weight represents excess water, since many patients in shock have a low level of albumin, resulting in a decrease in oncotic pressure (see paragraph headed "Albumin" on page 188).

Anthropometric measurement

Anthropometric measurements—including triceps skinfold (TSF), midarm circumference (MAC), and mid-upper-arm muscle circumference (MUAMC)—allow for the simple, quick identification of muscle depletion and loss of caloric reserves. (The measurements obtained are compared with standard values to determine the degree of depletion.) MAC is measured at the midpoint of the upper arm, halfway between the acromial process of the scapula and the olecranon process of the ulna. TSF, provides an estimate of the body's fat reserves, potentially a rich source of endogenous calories. It is measured at the midpoint of the nondominant upper arm. A fold of skin on the dorsal aspect is pulled away from the underlying muscle and measured with calipers. MUAMC is an indicator of the level of somatic protein deficit and is calculated from the values of MAC and TSF with the following equation:

$$\text{MUAMC} = \text{MAC} - (0.314 \times \text{TSF})$$

Deficits of less than 5% are insignificant; those between 5 and 15% are mild and point to recovery; deficits between 15 and 30% are serious and raise doubts about the patient's survival.

In summary, these measurements give important information concerning weight loss, fat stores, and the status of somatic protein as lean muscle mass.

Urinalysis

Creatinine. Analysis of urine specimens for creatinine can also help to indicate muscle status, since there is a linear relationship between the quantity of creatinine excreted and muscle mass. The creatinine/height index is calculated by first measuring the actual urinary creatinine for a 24-hour period and then comparing this with a standard. Stress can falsely elevate creatinine output and suggest that the somatic compartment is in better shape than it is.

Urea nitrogen. Figures on urinary urea nitrogen excreted over 24 hours are also helpful in estimating the actual metabolic expenditure and degree of hypermetabolism. When no protein is being ingested, stress—including that of infection—means the depletion of body energy stores; specifically, from 12 to 16% of the calorie expenditure is provided by the oxidation of amino acids. Urine urea nitrogen measurements are also needed for the determination and evaluation of therapy.

Other laboratory tests

Visceral protein level is assessed primarily through laboratory studies of albumin, transferrin, and total lymphocyte count.

Albumin. Albumin, a protein of hepatic origin, serves as a carrier for several molecules that require protein binding. Intravascular oncotic pressure is also highly dependent on albumin. If the hydrostatic pressure within a blood vessel is normal, an albumin above 2.8 g/dL is required to maintain relative dryness, thus preventing edema.

Transferrin. Transferrin, also a protein of hepatic origin, is smaller and more specific than albumin and is the protein that carries iron. A change in the level of transferrin will precede a change in albumin, since the former has a shorter half-life; therefore transferrin is a good indicator of muscle depletion and repair. If transferrin levels cannot be obtained, they can be derived from the total iron-binding capacity as follows:

$$\text{Serum transferrin} = \text{TIBC} \times 0.8 - 43$$

Lymphocytes. The total lymphocyte count (TLC) reflects the patient's immune status, since both T and B cells are included. TLC is calculated as follows:

$$\text{TLC} = \%\ \text{lymphocytes} \times \text{WBC}/100$$

The normal TLC is 2,000/mnu^3. Lymphopenia and failure of the immune system can arise from many acute or chronic causes, although they are often due to malnutrition.

Skin tests

Skin testing to determine a patient's response to common recall antigens should also be part of the overall nutritional assessment. Cell-mediated immunity is exemplified by the delayed type of hypersensitivity reaction in the skin. The principal effectors of this type of immunity are T cells that have become sensitized to foreign substances.

Positive reactions. When an individual has previously been sensitized to a particular antigen, its intradermal injection leads to a reaction of erythema followed by induration; this reaction reaches a peak in approximately 2 days. Lymphocytes and macrophages are the predominant cells in the lesion.

Negative reactions. Negative response to all antigens injected indicates anergy. Hospitalized patients demonstrating anergy have higher rates of sepsis and death than those with normal skin reactivity.

Malnourished patients are often anergic. When adequate nutritional support is provided, the immune response can return to normal. Certain diseases (such as immunodeficiency disorders) and the administration of some drugs (such as glucocorticoids) may also lead to negative skin reaction.

Treatment

Malnutrition in hospitalized patients is treated either by adequate dietary intake or by enteral or parenteral nutrition. The choice of therapy is based on the patient's general condition, the nutritional assessment, and the functioning of the GI tract.

GENERAL REFERENCES

Alpers D, Clouse R, Stenson W: *Manual of Nutritional Therapeutics*. Boston: Little, Brown, 1983

Blackburn G, Bistrian B, Maine B, et al: Nutritional and metabolic assessment of the hospitalized patient. *J Parenter Enter Nutr* 1:11, 1977

Ghadimi H: *Total Parenteral Nutrition: Premises and Promises*. New York: Wiley, 1975

Kaminski M, Ruggiero P: Nutritional assessment and support: Why, when, how? *Staff Phys* p 94, March 1980

Keithley J: Infection and the malnourished patient. *Heart Lung* 12:23, 1983

APPENDIX

DRUGS USED IN CRITICAL CARE

JACQUELINE M. CAROLAN, RN, BSN, CCRN

Drugs Used In Critical Care

DRUG	ACTION/INDICATIONS	DOSAGE	SIDE EFFECTS
Atropine sulfate	Reduces vagal tone, enhances AV conduction, increases heart rate Used to treat hemodynamically significant bradycardia and for temporary treatment of second- and third-degree heart block	0.5 to 2 mg by slow IV bolus	Paradoxical bradycardia may occur with doses below 0.25 mg Atrial and ventricular tachyarrhythmias, myocardial infarction from tachycardia and increased oxygen consumption
Bretylium tosylate (Bretylol)	Suppresses ventricular fibrillation rapidly and ventricular tachycardia and ectopy within 20 minutes to 2 hours. Has a positive inotropic effect on the myocardium Used for life-threatening ventricular arrhythmias that fail to respond to other antiarrhythmic therapy	5 mg/kg by rapid IV push for ventricular fibrillation; increased to 10 mg/kg every 15 to 30 minutes to maximum of 30 mg/kg. Continuous IV of 1 to 2 mg/min for treating other ventricular arrhythmias	Hypotension, increased frequency of arrhythmias, bradycardia

Calcium chloride	Increases myocardial contractility and tone, ventricular excitability, and conduction velocity through the ventricular muscle Used to improve myocardial contractility	250 to 500 mg slow IV bolus, repeated every 10 minutes as needed Precipitates in presence of sodium bicarbonate	Rapid administration may cause sinus bradycardia or arrest. Give cautiously to patients on digoxin
Dexamethasone sodium phosphate (Decadron)	Antiinflammatory, suppresses the immune system, and affects protein and carbohydrate metabolism Used to reduce cerebral edema and in pneumonias caused by aspiration or chemical irritants	4 to 8 mg IV or IM; therapy may continue until effect is achieved	Rare with short-term administration. Adrenal crisis if drug is discontinued abruptly
Digoxin (Lanoxin)	Increases myocardial contraction, slows heart rate and conduction through the AV node Used to control ventricular rate in atrial fibrillation, to treat paroxysmal tachycardia, and in congestive heart failure	0.5 to 0.75 mg slow IV push initially, followed by 0.25 mg slow IV push every 4 to 6 hours until maximum dosage or effect is achieved	Ventricular bigeminy, tachycardia, or fibrillation. AV dissociation, second- or third-degree heart block

DRUG	ACTION/INDICATIONS	DOSAGE	SIDE EFFECTS
Diphenhydramine hydrochloride (Benadryl)	Antihistamine, sedative; mild anticholinergic effect Used to treat allergic reactions and anaphylactic shock	25 to 50 mg IM or IV push	Drowsiness, incoordination, hypotension, palpitations
Dobutamine hydrochloride (Dobutrex)	Increases coronary artery and renal perfusion through increased cardiac output; promotes diuresis in patients with heart failure Used to treat cardiac decompensation caused by organic heart disease or cardiac surgery	2.5 to 10 μg/kg/min titrated to patient response (e.g., BP, heart rate, urine output, pulmonary artery wedge pressure, and cardiac output)	Increased heart rate and blood pressure. May precipitate ventricular ectopy

Dopamine hydrochloride (Intropin)	Effects vary with dosage Low dose: increased renal and coronary flow. May cause slight decrease in peripheral vascular resistance Medium dose: increased myocardial contractility, heart rate, stroke volume, and cardiac output. May increase peripheral resistance High dose: decreased renal blood flow, marked increase in peripheral vasoconstriction. Increased stroke volume, myocardial contractility, and cardiac output Used in treating hypotension (if volume replacement is adequate), cardiogenic shock secondary to left ventricular failure, and other shock states	Titrated to patient response Low: 2 to 5 μg/kg/min Medium: 5 to 30 μg/kg/min High: over 30 μg/kg/min	Tachyarrhythmias, increased myocardial oxygen consumption, myocardial ischemia

DRUG	ACTION/INDICATIONS	DOSAGE	SIDE EFFECTS
Epinephrine (Adrenalin)	Increases heart rate, myocardial contractility, systemic vascular resistance, arterial blood pressure, myocardial oxygen consumption, cardiac automaticity, and spontaneous ventricular contraction. Decreases defibrillation threshold Used to increase perfusion pressure in cardiac arrest, correct asystole and clinically significant bradyarrhythmias, and improve the efficacy of defibrillation	0.5 to 1 mg IV followed by 0.5 mg IV every 5 minutes as needed for cardiac arrest	Tachycardia, ventricular arrhythmias, myocardial ischemia and necrosis, ectopy
Furosemide (Lasix)	Increases sodium excretion by blocking its reabsorption in proximal and distal tubules and loop of Henle. Increases potassium excretion Used in congestive heart failure, to treat cerebral	20 to 100 mg IV bolus, may be given in increments of 10 mg at intervals	Volume depletion with hypotension, hypokalemia with arrhythmias, and hyperosmolality with neurologic abnormalities.

	edema following cardiac arrest, and for other conditions where diuresis is indicated		
Isoproterenol (Isuprel)	Increases heart rate, myocardial contractility, automaticity, myocardial oxygen consumption, venous return to the heart, and blood pressure secondary to improved cardiac output	2 to 20 μg/min IV of a 1 mg/500 mL solution	Tachyarrhythmias, especially if digitalis toxicity is present; myocardial ischemia and necrosis; ectopy
Lidocaine (Xylocaine)	Depresses myocardial irritability, reduces ventricular automaticity and ectopy, increases electrical stimulation threshold during diastole Used to suppress ventricular ectopy, increase effectiveness of defibrillation	1 mg/kg IV bolus stat, followed by continuous infusion of 1 to 4 mg/min	Nausea, vomiting, lethargy, paresthesia, tinnitus, disorientation, coma, seizures Decreased cardiac output, depressed myocardium ectopy, and slowed AV conduction with heart block and asystole
Nitroglycerin	Relaxes small-vessel smooth muscle, dilates arteries and capillaries, especially	25 to 200 mg mixed in 100 to 500 mL IV fluid. Titrate dose to patient response	Headache, dizziness, nausea, vomiting, tachycardia, palpitations, apprehension,

DRUG	ACTION/INDICATIONS	DOSAGE	SIDE EFFECTS
	coronary circulation. Decreases myocardial ischemia Used to control blood pressure in preoperative hypertensive patients, for treating angina pectoris, to produce controlled hypotension during surgical procedures, and for congestive heart failure associated with acute myocardial infarction		restlessness, muscle twitching, hypotension
Norepinephrine bitartrate, levarterenol (Levophed)	Increases systemic vascular resistance, BP, and coronary blood flow; widens pulse pressure. Decreases renal, mesenteric, hepatic, cerebral, and skeletal muscle blood flow through marked vasoconstriction Use to treat clinical shock	0.1 to 0.2 μg/kg/min continuous IV titrated to BP response, preferably 90 to 100 mm Hg systolic	Sinus bradycardia or high-degree heart block as reflex due to increased vagal tone. Hypertensive crisis with cardiac and neurologic effects Ischemia and necrosis from infiltration of drug into tissues Acute renal failure if drug use is prolonged

Procainamide (Pronestyl)	Depresses myocardial irritability, slows conduction through the atria, bundle of His, and ventricles Used in ventricular arrhythmias, atrial fibrillation, paroxysmal atrial tachycardia	25 to 50 mg/min IV as continuous infusion	Lowered BP with IV use, ventricular asystole or fibrillation, lupus syndrome
Propranolol (Inderal)	Slows AV conduction, is an antiarrhythmic, reduces heart rate and myocardial contractility Used to control heart rate in tachyarrhythmias. Reduces blood pressure and oxygen demand of the myocardium	IV push, 1 to 3 mg given slowly. Administration rate not to exceed 1 mg/min	Bradycardia, congestive heart failure, increased AV block, atrial insufficiency, nausea, vomiting, abdominal cramps
Sodium bicarbonate	Combines with free hydrogen ions to neutralize acid and restore pH of blood Used to treat significant metabolic acidosis, especially if secondary to cardiac arrest	1 ampoule IV every 10 minutes based on patient need and pH determination	Alkalosis from overcorrection of acidosis, aggravated left ventricular failure, hyperosmolarity

DRUG	ACTION/INDICATIONS	DOSAGE	SIDE EFFECTS
Sodium nitroprusside (Nipride)	Produces peripheral vasodilation. Rapid reduction of BP in hypertensive crisis	0.5 to 8 μg/kg/min, titrated to response	Hypotension and its effects, nausea, diaphoresis, restlessness, cyanide poisoning
Verapamil (Isoptin)	Reduces afterload, myocardial contractility, and peripheral vascular resistance. Slows AV conduction Used to convert paroxysmal supraventricular tachycardias rapidly	5 to 10 mg IV bolus over 2 minutes; repeat 10 mg IV in 30 minutes if response inadequate	Hypotension, bradycardia, tachycardia, nausea, headache, dizziness, abdominal discomfort

INDEX

*Italic page numbers refer to illustrations.

D

T

U

V

W

OTHER TITLES OF RELATED INTEREST FROM MEDICAL ECONOMICS BOOKS

Trauma Nursing
Edited by Virginia D. Cardona, RN, MS, CCRN
ISBN 0-87489-341-0

Managing the Critically Ill Effectively
Edited by Margaret Van Meter, RN
ISBN 0-87489-274-0

Critical Care Nursing Review and Self-Test
Billie C. Meador, RN, MSN, CCRN
ISBN 0-87489-300-3

Complete Guide to Cancer Nursing
Edited by Marjorie Beyers, RN, PhD,
June Werner, RN, MSN, CNAA, and
Suzanne Durburg, RN, BSN, MEd
ISBN 0-87489-294-5

Nurses' Guide to Neurosurgical Patient Care
Patricia Rauch Rhodes, RN, CNRN
ISBN 0-87489-223-6

Pediatric Nursing Policies, Procedures, and Personnel
Eileen M. Sporing, RN, MSN,
Mary K. Walton, RN, MSN, and
Charlotte E. Cady, RN, MSN
ISBN 0-87489-339-9

Understanding Medications: The Hows and Whys of Drug Therapy
Morton J. Rodman, PhD
ISBN 0-87489-252-X

RN Medication Tips
Sara J. White, RPh, and
Karin Williamson, RN
ISBN 0-87489-251-1

Giving Medications Correctly and Safely
Andrew J. Bartilucci, PhD, and
Jane M. Durgin, CIJ, RN, MS
ISBN 0-87489-216-3

How to Calculate Drug Dosages
Angela R. Pecherer, RN, and
Suzanne L. Venturo, RN
ISBN 0-87489-140-X

Manual for IV Therapy Procedures, Second Edition
Shila R. Channell, RN, PhD
ISBN 0-87489-370-4

A Guide to IV Admixture Compatibility, Third Edition
New England Deaconess Hospital, Boston
ISBN 0-87489-248-1

RN Nursing Assessment Series

- **The Well Adult**
  ISBN 0-87489-281-3
- **Respiratory Problems**
  ISBN 0-87489-282-1
- **Metabolic Problems**
  ISBN 0-87489-284-8
- **Gastrointestinal Problems**
  ISBN 0-87489-285-6
- **Genitourinary Problems**
  ISBN 0-87489-286-4

Neurologic Problems
ISBN 0-87489-287-2

Musculoskeletal Problems
ISBN 0-87489-288-0

Cardiovascular Problems
ISBN 0-87489-289-9

The Well Infant and Child
ISBN 0-87489-290-2

RN's Survival Sourcebook: Coping With Stress
Gloria Ferraro Donnelly, RN, MSN
ISBN 0-87489-299-6

RN's Sex Q & A: Candid Advice for You and Your Patients
Dorothy DeMoya, RN, MSN,
Armando DeMoya, MD, and
Howard Lewis
ISBN 0-87489-360-7

For information, write to:
MEDICAL ECONOMICS BOOKS
Oradell, New Jersey 07649
Or dial toll-free: 1-800-223-0581, ext. 2755
(Within the 201 area: 262-3030, ext. 2755)